THE VEGAN VANGUARD

Pioneering Recipes For Plant-Lovers

JEFFERY CHAPMAN

TABLE OF CONTENTS

INTRODUCTION

Welcome to "**The Vegan Vanguard**," a culinary odyssey that redefines the essence of plant-based eating. This book is not just a collection of recipes; it's a manifesto for a movement that champions compassion, sustainability, and a zest for vibrant, wholesome foods that nourish both the body and soul.

In these pages, you will find more than just meals; you will discover a new relationship with food. It's a journey that celebrates the abundance of the earth, offering dishes that are as nourishing as they are delightful. Each recipe is a testament to the fact that vegan cuisine can be rich, varied, and utterly delicious.

The Vegan Vanguard is about making conscious choices that resonate with our deepest values. It's about recognizing the power we hold in our hands every time we pick up a fork. This book invites you to join a revolution—one that starts in the kitchen and ripples out to touch the heart of humanity and the world we share.

As you turn these pages, you'll be introduced to flavors that astonish, textures that gratify, and aromas that transport you to fields, forests, and gardens bursting with life. You'll learn how to craft meals that are not only a feast for the senses but also kind to the planet and all its inhabitants.

This is not just about abstaining from animal products; it's about embracing a lifestyle that exudes positivity and health. It's about being part of a community that believes in doing good, feeling good, and spreading that goodness in waves of change.

So, let's raise our glasses (filled with freshly blended green smoothies, perhaps) to **The Vegan Vanguard**—the forefront of a culinary revolution where every bite is an act of love and each meal is a step towards creating a better world. Here's to the joy of vegan cooking, the celebration of life, and the bright future we build together with every delicious, plant-powered dish. Welcome aboard.

CHAPTER ONE

Introduction to Veganism: Why Choosing a Plant-Based Lifestyle Matters

In the quest for a healthier self and planet, the path of veganism shines as a beacon of hope and transformation. This lifestyle choice is a profound statement of personal ethics, environmental stewardship, and a commitment to fostering a compassionate world.

The essence of veganism transcends the mere exclusion of animal products from one's diet; it is a holistic approach to living that seeks to minimize harm and maximize kindness. It is a conscious decision to align one's actions with the values of respect for all living beings and the environment that sustains us.

The Health Perspective
From a health standpoint, a plant-based lifestyle is a powerful ally. A plethora of scientific studies have illuminated the benefits of a diet rich in fruits, vegetables, legumes, nuts, and seeds. Such a diet is not only

abundant in essential nutrients but also conducive to maintaining a healthy weight, reducing the risk of chronic diseases, and promoting longevity.

The human body thrives on the complex array of vitamins, minerals, antioxidants, and fiber that plants provide. By choosing veganism, individuals often report increased energy levels, clearer skin, and an overall sense of well-being. It is a testament to the body's innate ability to heal and flourish when nourished with whole, plant-based foods.

The Ethical Dimension
Ethically, veganism is a reflection of one's innermost convictions regarding the treatment of animals. It is a stand against the industrialized cruelty that pervades factory farming and a rejection of the notion that animals are mere commodities. Vegans understand that animals are sentient beings with the capacity to feel joy, pain, and fear, and they strive to protect these creatures from suffering.

By adopting a vegan lifestyle, individuals send a powerful message that the exploitation of

animals for food, clothing, or any other purpose
is unacceptable. It is a peaceful protest that
seeks to end the cycle of violence and pave
the way for a more humane society.

The Environmental Impact
Environmentally, the shift towards veganism is
perhaps one of the most impactful actions an
individual can take to combat climate change.
Animal agriculture is a significant contributor to
greenhouse gas emissions, deforestation,
water pollution, and the depletion of natural
resources. The production of plant-based
foods, on the other hand, generally requires
less water, land, and energy, making it a more
sustainable option.

Choosing a vegan lifestyle is a vote for the
planet, a choice that supports the preservation
of ecosystems, the conservation of biodiversity,
and the health of future generations. It is an
acknowledgment that our daily choices have
far-reaching consequences for the Earth and
its inhabitants.

The Social Aspect

Socially, veganism can be a unifying force that brings together people from diverse backgrounds around a common goal. It fosters a sense of community and shared purpose among those who are passionate about making a difference. Veganism often leads to increased awareness of other social justice issues, as it encourages individuals to consider the broader implications of their choices.

The vegan movement is inclusive, inviting everyone to participate in creating a kinder, more equitable world. It is a movement built on the belief that all beings deserve to live free from oppression and that we have the power to effect positive change through our actions.

Veganism is more than a diet; it is a way of life that embodies compassion, health, and responsibility. It is a journey that challenges us to rethink our relationship with the natural world and our fellow creatures. By choosing a plant-based lifestyle, we take a stand for what matters—our health, our ethics, and our planet.

As we forge ahead, let us do so with the spirit of the vegan vanguard, leading with our hearts and our plates, towards a future where all life is valued and respected. This is the essence of veganism, and this is why choosing a plant-based lifestyle matters.

1:1 The Power of Compassion: Personal Stories and Reflections on Empathy for Animals

Compassion is the heart's response to another's pain, a deep empathy that compels us to act, to alleviate suffering wherever we find it. When it comes to animals, this compassion takes on a profound significance. It becomes a bridge that connects us to the most innocent and vulnerable among us, urging us to consider their lives as valuable as our own.

The Silent Whispers of Empathy

Empathy for animals is often a whisper that grows louder with each encounter. It's in the gentle nudge of a dog seeking affection, the contented purr of a cat basking in the sun, or the curious gaze of a cow. These moments are the threads that weave the tapestry of compassion, revealing a shared desire for comfort, safety, and love.

For many, the journey towards empathy begins with personal stories—moments of connection that open our eyes to the rich emotional lives of animals. These narratives are powerful, for they speak of a recognition that animals, too, experience joy, sorrow, fear, and love. They remind us that animals are not mere objects or resources but sentient beings with their own perspectives on the world.

A Shift in Perspective
The realization that animals deserve our empathy often leads to a shift in perspective. It challenges us to look beyond our preconceived notions and to see animals as fellow travelers on this planet. This shift is not always easy; it requires us to confront uncomfortable truths about how our choices impact the lives of other creatures.

Yet, it is within this discomfort that growth occurs. As we begin to align our actions with our values, we find that our capacity for compassion expands. We start to advocate for animals, not because we have to, but because we understand their plight and recognize our ability to make a difference.

Stories of Transformation

The stories of those who have embraced this empathy are as varied as they are inspiring. There's the tale of the farmer who, upon recognizing the individual personalities of his cows, could no longer bear to send them to slaughter. Or the story of the fashionista who traded her fur coats for cruelty-free alternatives after learning of the suffering behind her luxury garments.

These stories are not just anecdotes; they are reflections of a growing consciousness that sees animal welfare as integral to a just society. They are evidence of a collective awakening to the idea that compassion for animals is not a sacrifice but a fulfillment of our most humane instincts.

The Role of Veganism

Veganism emerges as a natural extension of this empathy. It is a practical expression of compassion, a daily reaffirmation of our commitment to do no harm. By choosing plant-based foods, cruelty-free products, and entertainment that respects animal autonomy, we live out the principles of empathy in tangible ways.

Veganism is not about deprivation; it is about abundance—an abundance of kindness, health, and harmony. It is a celebration of life in all its forms and a recognition that we are all connected. When we choose veganism, we choose a path that honors the intrinsic value of every living being.

The Vanguard of Compassion
The Vegan Vanguard is a movement of individuals who lead with their hearts, who dare to imagine a world where compassion is the norm. It is a community of activists, thinkers, and dreamers who understand that empathy for animals is not a weakness but a strength.

As members of the Vegan Vanguard, we carry the torch of compassion, illuminating the darkness of indifference and cruelty. We share our stories, not to judge or condemn, but to inspire and educate. We lead by example, showing that a life of empathy is not only possible but deeply rewarding.

The power of compassion is immeasurable. It has the ability to transform hearts, change minds, and create a world where empathy for animals is woven into the fabric of society. As we share our personal stories and reflections, we contribute to a collective narrative of hope and change.

Let us continue to nurture this empathy, to spread the message of compassion far and wide. For in doing so, we uphold the spirit of the Vegan Vanguard, a force for good that champions the rights of all beings to live free from harm and suffering.

1:2 Your Vegan Manifesto: Crafting a Mission Statement for Your Vegan Journey

In the heart of every person who chooses the vegan way lies a manifesto, a declaration of intent, and a map of the heart's deepest convictions. This manifesto is not written in haste; it is a deliberate, thoughtful articulation of a commitment to a life lived with intention, kindness, and an unwavering dedication to the welfare of all living beings.

The Essence of Your Manifesto
Your manifesto is your voice in the chorus of change, a personal vow that resonates with the core principles of veganism. It is a reflection of your understanding that the choices we make at the dining table ripple out into the world, affecting ecosystems, societies, and countless lives.

Crafting your manifesto begins with introspection, a look inward to the values that guide your actions. It is an exploration of why you choose to stand against the tide, to live differently in a world that often seems indifferent to the suffering of animals and the degradation of our planet.

A Declaration of Compassion

At its core, your manifesto is a declaration of compassion. It is an acknowledgment that the ability to feel pain and desire happiness is not limited to humans but is shared by all creatures. Your manifesto is a pledge to honor that shared experience, to extend your circle of empathy to include every being that draws breath.

Compassion is the thread that weaves through every aspect of veganism, from the food we eat to the clothes we wear. It is a commitment to do no harm, to live in a way that minimizes suffering and maximizes kindness. Your manifesto is a testament to the belief that compassion is not a finite resource but an infinite wellspring that enriches our lives as we share it with others.

A Journey of Health and Harmony

Your manifesto also speaks to the pursuit of health and harmony, both within yourself and with the natural world. It celebrates the abundance of plant-based nutrition, the vitality that comes from eating foods that are as close to their natural state as possible.

This journey is not just about avoiding harm; it's about actively doing good—for your body, for animals, and for the planet. Your manifesto embraces the idea that health is not merely the absence of disease but a state of complete physical, mental, and social well-being.

A Stand for Sustainability
Your manifesto takes a stand for sustainability, recognizing that the current trajectory of human consumption is unsustainable. It is a call to action, urging us to rethink our relationship with the earth and its resources.

Sustainability is about more than just conservation; it's about regeneration—creating systems that replenish and restore. Your manifesto advocates for a lifestyle that supports this regenerative process, one that aligns with the rhythms of nature rather than seeking to dominate them.

A Vision of a Better World

Ultimately, your manifesto is a vision of a better world, a blueprint for a future where kindness reigns, and cruelty has no place. It is a dream of a society where every life is valued, where the rights of animals are respected, and where the health of the planet is a priority.

This vision is not a distant utopia; it is a world within our grasp. Your manifesto is a call to arms, inviting others to join you in creating this world, one choice, one meal, one act of kindness at a time.

Your Vegan Manifesto is more than words on a page; it is a living document, a guiding star on your journey towards a more compassionate, healthy, and sustainable life. It is a declaration of your values, a promise to yourself and the world, and a testament to the power of individual action to effect collective change.

As you craft your manifesto, let it be with passion, purpose, and the spirit of the Vegan Vanguard. Let it be a reflection of your unique voice, your story, and your vision for the future. And let it be a source of strength and inspiration as you walk the path of the vegan journey.

1:3 Vegan Pantry Essentials: Stocking Up on Must-Have Ingredients

Starting a vegan path makes the kitchen a creative and health-conscious haven. The cupboard transforms into a veritable gold mine of items that uplift the spirit and nourish the body. Stocking up on essential items ensures that you can always whip up something nutritious and delicious, embodying the spirit of the vegan vanguard with every meal.

Whole Grains: The Foundation of Vitality
Whole grains are the cornerstone of a well-stocked vegan pantry. Rich in fiber, vitamins, and minerals, they provide the energy needed to power through the day. Quinoa, brown rice, oats, and barley offer versatility and substance, serving as the base for a variety of dishes from hearty breakfasts to satisfying dinners.

Legumes: Protein-Packed Powerhouses

Legumes are the muscle behind the vegan diet, offering a hefty dose of protein essential for maintaining a healthy body. Black beans, lentils, chickpeas, and split peas are not only protein-rich but also brimming with fiber and iron. They can be transformed into soups, stews, salads, and even vegan burgers, proving that plant-based protein is both diverse and delectable.

Nuts and Seeds: Nutrient-Dense Nibbles

A selection of nuts and seeds is crucial for adding crunch and nutrition to any dish. Almonds, walnuts, chia seeds, and flaxseeds are packed with healthy fats, proteins, and omega-3 fatty acids. Sprinkle them on salads, blend them into smoothies, or create homemade nut butters—the possibilities are endless.

Herbs and Spices: The Essence of Flavor

Herbs and spices are the magic wands of the vegan kitchen, capable of transforming simple ingredients into culinary masterpieces. Stock up on basil, oregano, cumin, and turmeric to infuse your dishes with depth and complexity.

These flavor enhancers not only tantalize the taste buds but also boast a range of health benefits.

Condiments and Sauces: The Art of Accentuation

Condiments and sauces add the finishing touch to vegan dishes, elevating them from good to great. Tamari, apple cider vinegar, nutritional yeast, and plant-based milk are staples that lend richness and tang to recipes. Whether you're dressing a salad or creating a creamy sauce, these essentials are key to achieving the perfect balance of flavors.

Sweeteners: The Touch of Sweetness

In the world of vegan baking and dessert-making, natural sweeteners play a starring role. Maple syrup, coconut sugar, and dates offer a way to sweeten treats without resorting to refined sugars. They provide a subtle sweetness that complements rather than overpowers the natural flavors of your ingredients.

Plant-Based Proteins: The Meat Alternatives

For those times when you crave the texture and taste of meat, plant-based proteins come to the rescue. Tofu, tempeh, and seitan stand in as versatile alternatives that soak up flavors and provide a satisfying chew. Marinate them, grill them, or stir-fry them—their adaptability is a vegan's delight.

Canned Goods: The Convenience Factor

Canned goods are the unsung heroes of the vegan pantry, offering convenience without compromising on nutrition. Canned tomatoes, coconut milk, and pumpkin puree are just a few examples that can be the basis for soups, curries, and pies. Opt for low-sodium versions and BPA-free cans to keep your meals as healthy as they are convenient.

Superfoods: The Extra Boost

Superfoods like spirulina, goji berries, and cacao nibs might sound like the stuff of legend, but they're real and ready to elevate your health. These nutrient-packed ingredients can be sprinkled on oatmeal, blended into smoothies, or mixed into energy bars, giving you an extra boost of antioxidants and vitamins.

Creating a vegan pantry is about more than just stocking up on ingredients; it's about preparing for a lifestyle that is rich in health, flavor, and compassion. Each item on your shelf represents a choice—a choice to nourish yourself, to protect animals, and to tread lightly on the earth.

As you fill your pantry with these essentials, remember that each ingredient is a building block for a meal that upholds the values of the vegan vanguard. With passion, purpose, and a pantry full of plant-based power, you are equipped to craft dishes that are not only good for you but also good for the world.

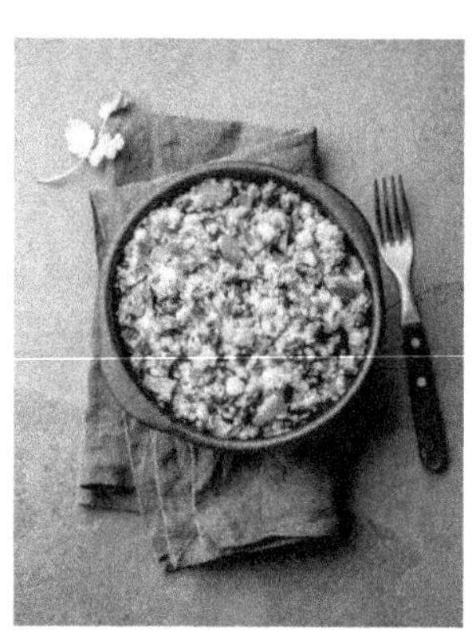

Quinoa and Black Bean Salad

CHAPTER TWO

Fueling the Revolution: A Call to Action for the Vegan Vanguard

The revolution is not just fought on the streets; it is also fought in the kitchens, in the grocery stores, and on the dining tables of the world. It is a revolution of consciousness, a collective awakening to the impact of our food choices on the planet, on animals, and on our health. This revolution is fueled not by anger or violence, but by love, compassion, and the unwavering belief in a better future—a future that is possible through the power of veganism.

The Vegan Vanguard: Pioneers of Change

The Vegan Vanguard is a growing force, a community of pioneers leading the charge towards this brighter future. These are the individuals who understand that every meal is a statement of intent, an opportunity to stand up for what is right and just. They are the ones who recognize that the simple act of choosing plant-based foods is a radical act of kindness and sustainability.

The Role of Food: Nourishment and Connection

Food is the fuel that powers the revolution, and it is so much more than mere sustenance. It is a source of connection, a way to share our values and our hopes with others. Vegan food is a celebration of life, bursting with flavors, colors, and textures that delight the senses and nourish the body.

The dishes we create and share are expressions of our commitment to non-violence and our respect for all living beings. They are proof that compassion can be delicious, that there is joy in simplicity, and that abundance does not require sacrifice.

Education and Advocacy: Spreading the Word

Fueling the revolution also involves education and advocacy. It is about sharing knowledge, dispelling myths, and opening hearts and minds to the benefits of a vegan lifestyle. The Vegan Vanguard is at the forefront of this educational mission, armed with facts, stories, and an infectious enthusiasm for change.

Through cooking classes, workshops, books, and social media, the message is spreading. People are learning about the health benefits of a plant-based diet, the ethical implications of animal agriculture, and the environmental necessity of reducing our reliance on animal products.

Community and Support: Building a Movement

No revolution can succeed without a strong community, and the Vegan Vanguard is all about building connections and offering support. It is a movement that thrives on inclusivity, welcoming everyone, regardless of where they are on their vegan journey.

Support comes in many forms, from potlucks and meetups to online forums and mentorship programs. It is about creating a space where questions are encouraged, challenges are met with empathy, and successes are celebrated together.

Innovation and Creativity: The Vegan Economy

The revolution is also driving innovation and creativity, giving rise to a burgeoning vegan economy. New businesses are emerging, offering plant-based alternatives to traditional animal products. These range from dairy-free cheeses and meatless burgers to cruelty-free clothing and sustainable beauty products.

The Vegan Vanguard supports these enterprises, understanding that a strong vegan economy is essential for the longevity of the movement. By choosing to spend their money on vegan products and services, they are helping to create a market that reflects their values.

Activism and Policy: Shaping the Future

Activism is another crucial component of fueling the revolution. Members of the Vegan Vanguard are not content to simply live their values; they are also determined to effect change on a larger scale. This involves everything from peaceful protests and letter-writing campaigns to lobbying for policy changes that promote plant-based living.

The goal is to create a world where vegan options are accessible to everyone, where animal rights are recognized and protected, and where the environment is treated with the care it deserves.

Fueling the revolution is about so much more than what we eat. It is about who we are and the world we want to create. It is a call to action for all those who believe in the power of compassion, the importance of health, and the urgency of environmental stewardship.

The Vegan Vanguard is leading the way, showing that a different way of living is not only possible but also joyful and fulfilling. With every plant-based meal, every educational conversation, and every act of advocacy, they are fueling a revolution that has the power to transform the world.

Let us join them, with passion, purpose, and the spirit of the Vegan Vanguard, as we work together to create a future that is kinder, healthier, and more sustainable for all.

2:1 Plant-Powered Nutrition: Understanding Essential Nutrients and Meal Planning

In the vibrant world of veganism, nutrition is the canvas, and plants are the palette with which we paint our healthiest selves. This chapter delves into the essential nutrients that are the keystones of vitality and provides a guide to crafting meal plans that are as nourishing as they are delightful. Accompanied by recipes that are both simple to prepare and bursting with flavor, this is your guide to thriving on a plant-based diet.

Essential Nutrients for a Thriving Vegan
A well-planned vegan diet is rich in essential nutrients, each playing a unique role in maintaining optimal health. Proteins, carbohydrates, fats, vitamins, and minerals come together in a symphony of nourishment that supports every function of the body.

Proteins are essential for tissue growth and repair, serving as the building blocks of life.

Legumes, nuts, seeds, and whole grains are excellent sources of plant-based protein that can easily meet and exceed your daily requirements.

Carbohydrates are the body's primary energy source, fueling everything from brain function to physical activity. Whole grains, fruits, and vegetables provide complex carbohydrates, fiber, and a host of phytonutrients that promote sustained energy and digestive health.

In order to produce hormones, maintain a healthy brain, and absorb fat-soluble vitamins, one must consume fats. Avocados, nuts, seeds, and plant oils offer healthy unsaturated fats, including omega-3 fatty acids, which are crucial for heart health and cognitive function.

Vitamins and minerals are the micronutrients that catalyze and regulate bodily processes. A colorful array of fruits and vegetables ensures a rich intake of these nutrients, with dark leafy greens, berries, and citrus fruits being particularly nutrient-dense.

Meal Planning for Success

Meal planning is the art of orchestrating your nutrient intake to support your health goals. It involves selecting a variety of foods that provide a balance of macronutrients and micronutrients to keep you energized and satisfied throughout the day.

Start by planning your meals around a protein source, adding a variety of vegetables and a whole grain or starchy vegetable for a complete meal. Snacks can include fresh fruit, vegetable sticks with hummus, or a handful of nuts and seeds.

Recipes to Ignite Your Culinary Passion

Let's explore some recipes that embody the essence of plant-powered nutrition, each a celebration of flavor and health.

Quinoa and Black Bean Salad

Ingredients:

1 cup quinoa

2 cups water

1 can black beans, drained and rinsed

1 red bell pepper, diced

1/4 cup fresh cilantro, chopped

Juice of 1 lime

2 tablespoons olive oil

Salt and pepper to taste

Instructions:
1. Rinse the quinoa under cold water. Bring the water and quinoa to a boil in a pot. Reduce heat, cover, and simmer for 15 minutes until the quinoa is fluffy.
2. In a large bowl, combine the cooked quinoa, black beans, red bell pepper, and cilantro.
3. Combine the olive oil, lime juice, salt, and pepper in a small bowl. After pouring, toss the salad to mix.
4. Serve chilled or at room temperature.

Creamy Avocado Pasta
Ingredients:
12 oz whole wheat pasta

2 ripe avocados, pitted and peeled

2 cloves garlic

2 tablespoons lemon juice

1/3 cup olive oil

Salt and pepper to taste

Cherry tomatoes and basil for garnish

Instructions:
1. Cook pasta according to package
instructions. Drain and set aside.
2. In a food processor, blend avocados, garlic,
lemon juice, and olive oil until smooth.
3. Toss the pasta with the avocado sauce.
Season with salt and pepper.
4. Garnish with cherry tomatoes and fresh basil
before serving.

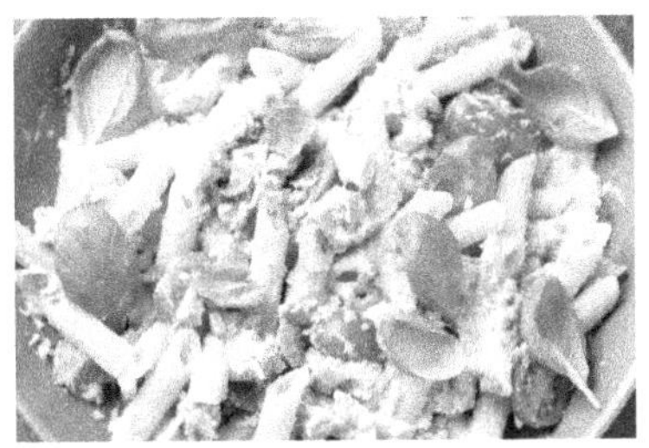

Creamy Avocado Pasta

Tips for Meal Preparation
Batch Cooking: Prepare grains and legumes in bulk at the beginning of the week to save time on busy days.
Freshness First: Prioritize fresh produce to maximize nutrient intake and flavor.
Seasonal Selections: Choose seasonal fruits and vegetables for the best taste and nutritional value.
Spice It Up: Don't shy away from herbs and spices; they can transform a dish while adding minimal calories.

Choosing a plant-based diet is an educational process, a path that leads to a deeper understanding of the food we eat and its impact on our bodies and the world. With the right knowledge and a collection of enticing recipes, anyone can craft a vegan diet that is as satisfying as it is healthful.

Let this be your manifesto, a declaration of your commitment to nourishing your body with the finest ingredients nature has to offer. Let each meal be a step towards a healthier you and a more compassionate world. This is the spirit of the Vegan Vanguard, and it begins with what we put on our plates.

2:2 Protein Powerhouses: Delicious High-Protein Vegan Recipes

In the vibrant landscape of vegan cuisine, protein-rich dishes stand tall as the pillars of nourishment and satisfaction. This chapter is a celebration of plant-based proteins, showcasing recipes that are not only packed with nutritional value but also brimming with flavors that will tantalize your taste buds. Each recipe is a testament to the versatility and abundance that vegan cooking offers, proving that a diet rich in plants can fulfill all your protein needs.

The Mighty Legume: Chickpea Salad Bowl
Chickpeas, also known as garbanzo beans, are a staple in the vegan pantry. They are versatile, delicious, and a fantastic source of protein. This chickpea salad bowl is a perfect example of how simple ingredients can come together to create a meal that is both satisfying and nutritious.

Ingredients:
2 cups cooked chickpeas

1 large cucumber, diced

1 red bell pepper, diced

1/4 cup red onion, finely chopped

1/4 cup fresh parsley, chopped

2 tablespoons olive oil

Juice of 1 lemon

Salt and pepper to taste

Instructions:
1. In a large bowl, combine the chickpeas, cucumber, bell pepper, red onion, and parsley.
2. Drizzle with olive oil and lemon juice, then season with salt and pepper.
3. Toss everything together until well mixed.
4. Serve immediately or let it chill in the refrigerator for an hour to allow the flavors to meld.

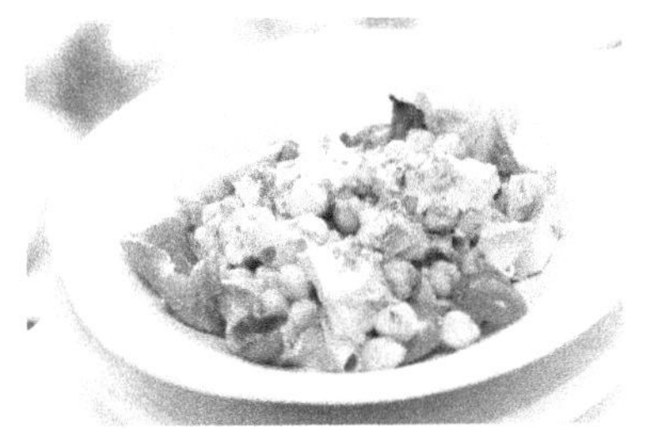

Chickpea Salad

The Seed of Life: Quinoa Stuffed Peppers
Quinoa is a true superfood, a complete protein containing all nine essential amino acids. These quinoa stuffed peppers are not only protein-packed but also filled with a rainbow of nutrients from various vegetables.

Ingredients:
4 large bell peppers, halved and seeds removed

1 cup quinoa, cooked

1 can of washed and drained black beans

1 cup corn kernels

1/2 cup tomatoes, diced

1 teaspoon cumin

1 teaspoon paprika

1/2 teaspoon garlic powder

Salt and pepper to taste

1/4 cup vegan cheese, shredded (optional)

Instructions:
1. Preheat your oven to 375°F (190°C).
2. In a bowl, mix together the cooked quinoa, black beans, corn, tomatoes, cumin, paprika, and garlic powder. Season with salt and pepper.
3. Stuff each bell pepper half with the quinoa mixture and place in a baking dish.
4. Top with vegan cheese if using.
5. Cover with foil and bake for 25 minutes. Remove the foil and bake for another 10 minutes until the peppers are tender and the tops are slightly browned.

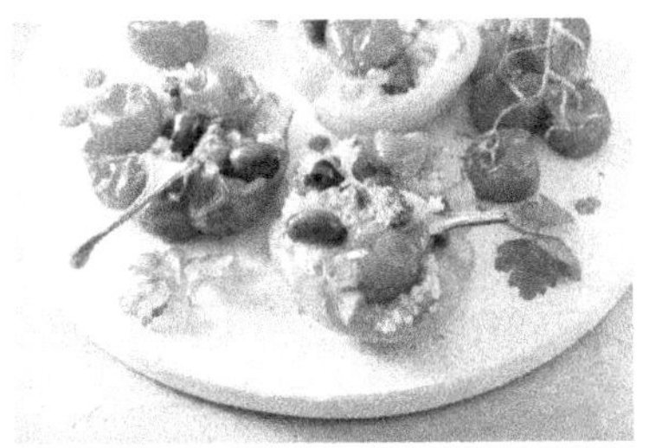

Stuffed Peppers

The Nutty Affair: Almond Butter Tofu Stir-Fry

Tofu is a beloved protein source in the vegan world. When paired with almond butter, it creates a stir-fry that is rich in protein and flavor.

Ingredients:
14 oz firm tofu, pressed and cubed

2 tablespoons soy sauce

2 tablespoons almond butter

1 tablespoon maple syrup

1 tablespoon rice vinegar

1 teaspoon sesame oil

1 tablespoon olive oil

2 cups of mixed veggies, such as carrots, snap peas, broccoli, and bell peppers

- Sesame seeds for garnish

Instructions:
1. In a bowl, whisk together soy sauce, almond butter, maple syrup, rice vinegar, and sesame oil until smooth.
2. In a pan set over medium heat, warm the olive oil. Tofu cubes should be added and cooked until golden brown all over.
3. Add the mixed vegetables to the pan and stir-fry until they are tender-crisp.
4. Pour the almond butter sauce over the tofu and vegetables, stirring to coat everything evenly.
5. Cook for another 2-3 minutes until the sauce is heated through.
6. Garnish with sesame seeds before serving.

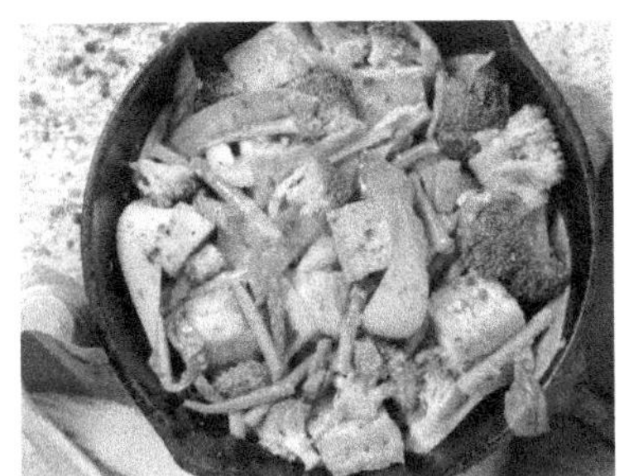

Tofu and vegetables Stir-Fry

Tips for High-Protein Vegan Cooking

Embrace Variety: Incorporate a range of protein sources in your diet to ensure you're getting a complete profile of amino acids.

Plan Ahead: Prepare protein-rich components like beans and grains in advance to make meal prep quicker and easier.

Get Creative: Use herbs and spices to add depth and excitement to your dishes without the need for high-sodium sauces.

Balance Your Plate: Pair protein-rich foods with a variety of vegetables and healthy fats for a well-rounded meal.

These recipes are just a glimpse into the world of high-protein vegan cooking. Each dish is crafted with care, ensuring that every bite is as nourishing as it is delicious. As you explore these recipes, let them inspire you to create your own protein-packed meals, fueling your body with the best that plant-based eating has to offer.

Remember, the journey to a healthier, more compassionate life is paved with the foods we choose to eat. Let these protein powerhouses be your companions on this journey, providing the strength and vitality needed to carry the torch of the Vegan Vanguard.

2:3 Superfood Spotlight: Exploring Nutrient-Rich Ingredients

In the realm of health and wellness, superfoods are the celebrated heroes, offering a myriad of benefits in each vibrant bite. These nutrient-rich ingredients are the stars of the vegan diet, providing a wealth of vitamins, minerals, antioxidants, and more. This chapter is dedicated to these powerful foods, exploring their benefits and showcasing how they can be incorporated into delicious, healthful recipes that align with the spirit of the Vegan Vanguard.

Chia Seeds: Tiny Titans of Nutrition

Chia seeds are small in size but mighty in nutrition. Packed with omega-3 fatty acids, fiber, and protein, they are an excellent addition to any meal. Their ability to absorb water and form a gel-like consistency makes them a versatile ingredient in vegan cooking.

Chia Seed Pudding

Ingredients:

1/4 cup chia seeds

1 cup unsweetened almond milk

1 tablespoon maple syrup

1/2 teaspoon vanilla extract

Fresh berries for topping

Instructions:
1. In a bowl, mix chia seeds with almond milk, maple syrup, and vanilla extract.
2. Stir well and let sit for 5 minutes. Stir again to break up any clumps.
3. Refrigerate for a minimum of two hours or overnight while covered.
4. Serve topped with fresh berries.

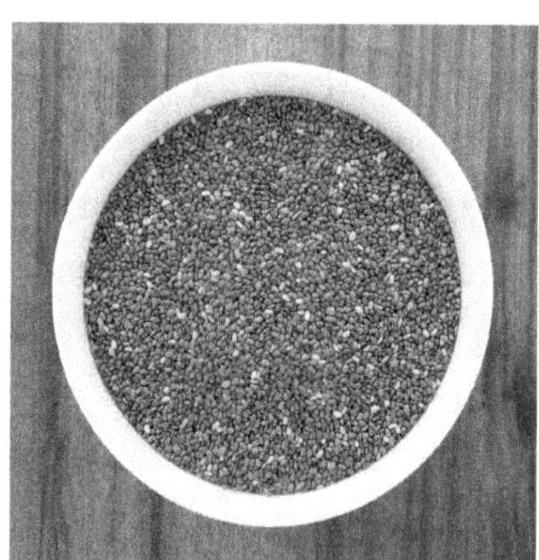

Chia Seeds

Kale: The Leafy Green Superstar

Kale is a leafy green that has gained fame for its dense nutritional profile. It has a lot of calcium, iron, and the vitamins A, C, and K. Kale can be enjoyed raw, sautéed, or baked into crispy chips.

Garlicky Sautéed Kale

Ingredients:

1 bunch kale, stems removed and leaves chopped

2 cloves garlic, minced

1 tablespoon olive oil

Salt and pepper to taste

Lemon wedges for serving

Instructions:

1. In a big pan set over medium heat, warm up the olive oil.
2. Add garlic and sauté until fragrant.
3. Add kale and cook until wilted and tender, about 5 minutes.
4. Season with salt and pepper.
5. Add some freshly squeezed lemon juice and serve.

Quinoa: The Complete Protein
Quinoa has all nine of the essential amino acids, making it a complete protein. It's also high in fiber and minerals like magnesium and manganese. Quinoa is a fantastic base for salads, bowls, and even breakfast dishes.

Quinoa Breakfast Bowl
Ingredients:
1/2 cup quinoa, rinsed

1 cup water
1 apple, diced

1/4 teaspoon cinnamon

1 tablespoon almond butter

A handful of walnuts, chopped

Instructions:
1. In a pot, combine quinoa and water. Bring to a boil, then reduce heat and simmer for 15 minutes until quinoa is cooked and water is absorbed.
2. Stir in diced apple and cinnamon.
3. Top with a dollop of almond butter and a sprinkle of chopped walnuts.

Berries: Nature's Candy
Berries are very nutrient-dense in addition to being delicious. They are high in fiber, vitamin C, and antioxidants known as anthocyanins. Berries can be eaten fresh, frozen, or dried, and they add a natural sweetness to any dish.

Mixed Berry Smoothie
Ingredients:
1 cup of mixed berries, including raspberries, blueberries, and strawberries

1 banana

1 cup spinach

1 cup unsweetened almond milk

1 tablespoon flax seeds

Instructions:
1. Combine all ingredients in a blender.
2. Blend until smooth.
3.Enjoy right away after pouring into a glass.

Tips on how to Superfoods into Your Diet

Start Small: Introduce new superfoods into your diet one at a time.
Mix and Match: Combine different superfoods to maximize their health benefits.
Get Creative: Use superfoods in a variety of dishes, from smoothies to soups to desserts.
Keep It Colorful: Aim for a rainbow of colors on your plate to ensure a diverse intake of nutrients.

Superfoods are a testament to the power of plant-based nutrition. They offer a simple yet profound way to enhance our health and vitality. By incorporating these nutrient-rich ingredients into our meals, we not only nourish our bodies but also support the principles of the Vegan Vanguard—living with passion, purpose, and a deep respect for all life.

As you explore the world of superfoods, let each recipe be an adventure, a chance to discover the flavors and benefits that these ingredients offer. With each superfood you embrace, you're taking a step towards a healthier, more vibrant life, fueling the revolution with every plant-powered bite.

2:4 Energizing Smoothies and Juices: Boosting Vitality with Liquid Nutrition

In the bustling rhythm of modern life, finding the time to nourish our bodies can be a challenge. Smoothies and juices offer a swift and delightful solution, packing a punch of nutrients in every sip. This chapter is a homage to these liquid elixirs of life, each recipe crafted to invigorate the body, awaken the senses, and support the vibrant lifestyle that is the hallmark of the Vegan Vanguard.

The Green Machine: A Symphony of Vitality
The Green Machine smoothie is a concoction designed to energize and detoxify. It's a blend of leafy greens and fruits, creating a balance of sweetness and nutrition that will leave you feeling refreshed and ready to take on the day.

Ingredients:
1 cup fresh spinach

1 cup kale leaves

1 ripe banana
1/2 green apple, cored and sliced

1 tablespoon chia seeds

1 cup coconut water

Ice cubes (optional)

Instructions:
1. Place the spinach, kale, banana, apple, and chia seeds in a blender.
2. Add coconut water and ice cubes if desired for a colder beverage.
3. Process on high until creamy and smooth..
4. Pour into a glass and enjoy immediately for the best taste and nutrient retention.

The Berry Bliss: Antioxidant-Rich Indulgence

Berries are nature's jewels, rich in antioxidants and bursting with flavor. The Berry Bliss is a smoothie that combines a variety of berries with the creaminess of almond milk, resulting in a drink that's as pleasing to the palate as it is beneficial for health.

Ingredients:

1 cup of mixed berries, comprising blueberries, raspberries, and strawberries

1 ripe banana

1 tablespoon ground flaxseed

1 cup unsweetened almond milk

An optional extra drop of agave syrup for sweetness

Instructions:
1. Add the mixed berries, banana, ground flaxseed, and almond milk to a blender.
2. Blend until smooth, adding agave syrup if a sweeter taste is desired.
3. Serve immediately, garnished with a few whole berries on top for a visually appealing presentation.

The Tropical Twist: A Zest for Life
The Tropical Twist juice is a vibrant blend of citrus and tropical fruits, designed to awaken your senses and provide a burst of vitamin C. This juice is perfect for those mornings when you need an extra zing to start your day.

Ingredients:
1 orange, peeled and quartered

1/2 cup pineapple chunks

1/2 mango, peeled and pitted

1/2 lime, juiced

1/2 inch piece of ginger, peeled

1/2 cup coconut water

Instructions:
1. Run the orange, pineapple, mango, and ginger through a juicer.
2. Stir in the lime juice and coconut water.
3. Serve chilled, over ice if preferred, for a refreshing tropical experience.

The Protein Punch: Fuel for the Active Soul
For those who lead an active lifestyle, the Protein Punch smoothie is the perfect post-workout refreshment. Combining plant-based protein powder with the natural sweetness of dates and bananas, this smoothie is both a treat and a muscle-recovery aid.

Ingredients:
1 ripe banana

2 Medjool dates, pitted

1 tablespoon natural peanut butter

1 scoop vegan protein powder (vanilla or chocolate)

1 cup soy milk

Ice cubes (optional)

Instructions:
1. Place the banana, dates, peanut butter, protein powder, and soy milk in a blender.
2. Add ice cubes if a thicker, colder smoothie is desired.
3. Blend until smooth and creamy.
4. Pour into a shaker bottle or glass and enjoy after your workout for optimal recovery.

Tips for Crafting the Perfect Smoothie or Juice

Fresh is Best: Use fresh, ripe fruits and vegetables to ensure maximum flavor and nutrient content.

Balance Your Ingredients: Combine a good mix of greens, fruits, and proteins to create a well-rounded drink.

Experiment with Superfoods: Add superfoods like spirulina, maca powder, or acai for an extra nutrient boost.

Mind the Sweetness: Be cautious with added sweeteners; let the natural sweetness of the fruits shine through.

Smoothies and juices are more than just beverages; they are a lifestyle choice that reflects a commitment to health and vitality. Each recipe in this collection is designed to support the principles of the Vegan Vanguard, offering a delicious way to fuel your body and spirit with the goodness of plants.

As you blend and juice your way through these recipes, let them be a daily reminder of the power of plant-based nutrition. Let them energize your body, delight your taste buds, and inspire you to live each day with passion, purpose, and the spirit of the Vegan Vanguard.

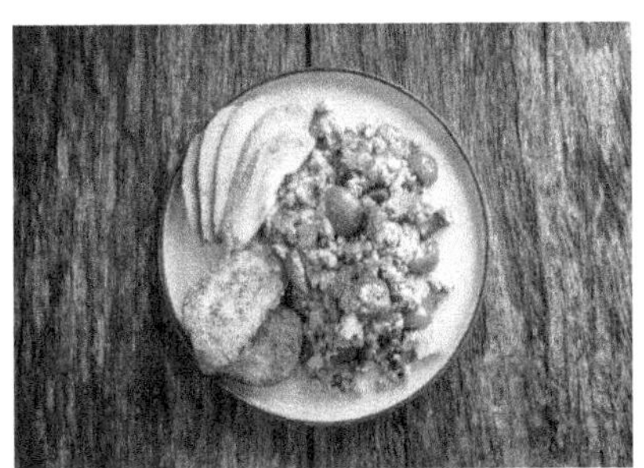

Scrabble Tofu

CHAPTER THREE

Culinary Warriors Unite: The Vanguard of Vegan Victuals

In the heart of every kitchen where compassion meets creativity, a culinary warrior stands, whisk in hand, ready to transform the bounty of the earth into a feast for the senses. This is the Vegan Vanguard, a brigade of brave souls who wield spatulas and knives in the name of health, sustainability, and animal welfare. They are the pioneers on the frontlines of the food revolution, crafting dishes that are as kind to the palate as they are to the planet.

The Vanguard's Creed

The culinary warriors of the Vegan Vanguard live by a creed that is simple yet profound: to create food that nourishes, delights, and inspires. They believe that cooking is an act of love—a love for life, for those who share their table, and for the world that provides their sustenance. Their kitchen is their sanctuary, and their recipes are their hymns of gratitude and respect.

The Arsenal of Ingredients

The Vegan Vanguard's arsenal is stocked with the freshest, most vibrant ingredients. Vegetables, fruits, legumes, grains, nuts, and seeds are their ammunition against the mundane and the mediocre. Each ingredient is chosen with care, ensuring that it meets the highest standards of quality and ethics.

Recipes for Revolution

The recipes that follow are more than mere instructions; they are blueprints for a better world. Each one is infused with the passion, purpose, and spirit that define the Vegan Vanguard.

Majestic Mushroom Bourguignon

A dish that pays homage to the classic French stew, this mushroom bourguignon is a hearty and satisfying centerpiece for any meal.

Ingredients:
2 tablespoons olive oil

4 cups cremini mushrooms, quartered

1 large onion, diced

2 carrots, sliced

2 cloves garlic, minced

1 cup red wine

2 cups vegetable broth

2 tablespoons tomato paste

1 teaspoon thyme

2 tablespoons of water and 1 tablespoon of cornstarch

Salt and pepper to taste

Fresh parsley for garnish

Instructions:
1. In a big pot, warm up the olive oil over medium heat. Cook the mushrooms until they turn golden brown.
2. Add onion, carrots, and garlic, cooking until softened.
3. Pour in red wine, scraping any bits off the bottom of the pot.
4. Stir in vegetable broth, tomato paste, and thyme. Bring to a simmer.

5. Add the cornstarch mixture, stirring until the sauce thickens.
6. Season with salt and pepper. Garnish with fresh parsley before serving.

Triumphant Tofu Scramble
Start your day with a protein-packed scramble that's as colorful as it is nutritious.

Ingredients:
1 brick of firm tofu, crushed and drained

1 tablespoon nutritional yeast

1/2 teaspoon turmeric

1/2 teaspoon paprika

1/4 cup plant milk

1/2 red bell pepper, diced

1/2 cup spinach, chopped

Salt and pepper to taste

Avocado slices for serving

Instructions:
1. In a bowl, mix crumbled tofu with nutritional yeast, turmeric, paprika, and plant milk.
2. Heat a non-stick pan over medium heat. Add the tofu mixture and cook for 5 minutes.
3. Stir in bell pepper and spinach, cooking until the vegetables are tender.
4. Season with salt and pepper. Serve with avocado slices on top.

Tips for the Aspiring Culinary Warrior
Stay Curious: Always be on the lookout for new ingredients and techniques to expand your culinary repertoire.
Embrace Simplicity: Sometimes the simplest dishes are the most profound. Allow the tastes of your components to come through naturally.
Cook with Intention: Remember that every dish you create is a reflection of your values and vision for a kinder world.

The Vegan Vanguard is more than a group of individuals; it is a movement, a collective force that is reshaping the way we think about food. As culinary warriors, we have the power to make a difference with every meal we prepare and every bite we take.

Let us unite in our kitchens, armed with our blenders and bowls, our pots and pans, to create a revolution that is delicious, nutritious, and compassionate. Let us cook with conviction, eat with enthusiasm, and live with purpose. For we are the Vegan Vanguard, and our time is now.

3:1 Global Gastronomy: Traveling the World Through Vegan Cuisine

The world is a mosaic of cultures, each with its own unique flavors, ingredients, and culinary traditions. Vegan cuisine, with its emphasis on plant-based ingredients, offers a passport to this global tapestry of tastes without ever leaving the kitchen. This journey through vegan gastronomy celebrates the diversity of global cuisines while adhering to the compassionate principles of the Vegan Vanguard.

A Feast of Flavors

Vegan cuisine is not confined by borders; it is a global affair that embraces the essence of each region's gastronomic delights. From the aromatic spices of India to the robust flavors of the Mediterranean, plant-based dishes can transport you to far-off lands.

The Indian Odyssey: Aromatic and Spicy

Indian cuisine is renowned for its intricate use of spices and herbs, creating dishes that are rich in flavor and aroma. The following recipe is a vegan twist on a classic Indian dish, bringing the essence of India to your dining table.

Chana Masala
Ingredients:
2 cups cooked chickpeas

1 large onion, finely chopped

2 tomatoes, pureed

2 cloves garlic, minced

1 inch ginger, grated

1 green chili, finely chopped

1 teaspoon cumin seeds

1 teaspoon ground coriander

1 teaspoon garam masala

1/2 teaspoon turmeric powder

1/2 teaspoon paprika

Salt to taste

2 tablespoons vegetable oil

Fresh cilantro for garnish

Instructions:
1. Heat oil in a pan and add cumin seeds. Once they start to sizzle, add onions and cook until golden brown.
2. Add garlic, ginger, and green chili. Sauté for a couple of minutes.
3. Stir in the tomato puree and cook until the oil separates from the mixture.
4. Add the spices—coriander, garam masala, turmeric, paprika, and salt. Cook for another minute.
5. Add the cooked chickpeas and enough water to make a thick gravy. Simmer for 10 minutes.
6. Serve over naan or rice with a fresh cilantro garnish.

The Mediterranean Voyage: Fresh and Wholesome

The Mediterranean diet is celebrated for its health benefits and its focus on fresh vegetables, fruits, and grains. The following recipe encapsulates the sunny flavors of the

Mediterranean in a dish that is both simple and sublime.

Mediterranean Quinoa Salad
Ingredients:
1 cup quinoa, cooked

1 cucumber, diced

1 bell pepper, diced

1/2 red onion, finely chopped

1/4 cup kalamata olives, sliced

1/4 cup sun-dried tomatoes, chopped

1/4 cup parsley, chopped

Juice of 1 lemon

2 tablespoons olive oil

Salt and pepper to taste

Instructions:
1. In a large bowl, combine the cooked quinoa, cucumber, bell pepper, red onion, olives, sun-dried tomatoes, and parsley.

2. Mix the olive oil, lemon juice, salt, and pepper in a small bowl.

3. Toss to mix after adding the dressing to the salad..

4. Chill in the refrigerator for at least 30 minutes before serving to allow the flavors to meld.

The Latin American Expedition: Vibrant and Hearty

Latin American cuisine is a celebration of bold flavors and hearty ingredients. The following recipe is a vegan version of a traditional Latin American dish, full of color and zest.

Black Bean and Sweet Potato Tacos

Ingredients:

2 sweet potatoes, peeled and diced

1 can of washed and drained black beans

1 avocado, sliced

1/2 red cabbage, shredded

1 lime, cut into wedges

8 corn tortillas

1 teaspoon chili powder

1/2 teaspoon cumin

Salt to taste

2 tablespoons vegetable oil

Instructions:
1. Preheat the oven to 400°F (200°C).
2. Toss sweet potatoes with oil, chili powder, cumin, and salt. Spread on a baking sheet and roast for 25 minutes until tender.
3. Warm the tortillas in the oven or on a skillet.
4. Assemble the tacos by placing a scoop of sweet potatoes and black beans on each tortilla.
5. Top with shredded cabbage and avocado slices.
6. Serve with lime wedges on the side.

Culinary Tips for the Global Vegan Chef
Explore Local Markets: Discover new ingredients and produce that are staples in different cuisines.

Experiment with Spices: Spices are the soul of many dishes.
Learn Traditional Techniques: Research and practice traditional cooking methods to add authenticity to your dishes.

Vegan cuisine is a boundless adventure, a way to explore the world's cultures through the universal language of food. Each recipe is a journey, an opportunity to learn, to taste, and to share. As members of the Vegan Vanguard, we unite under the banner of global gastronomy, celebrating the rich tapestry of flavors that our world has to offer.

Let us continue to cook with curiosity, to dine with delight, and to live with a passion for the diverse and delicious world of vegan cuisine. For in every bite lies the potential to connect, to understand, and to savor the beauty of our global community.

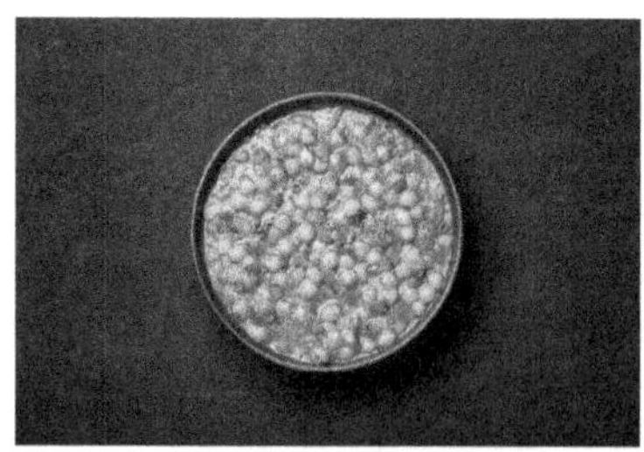

Chana Masala

3:2 Bold and Beautiful Bowls: Vibrant One-Bowl Meals

In the vibrant world of vegan cuisine, the bowl has become a canvas for culinary artists, a vessel where colors, textures, and flavors meld in harmonious symphony. These one-bowl meals are not just a feast for the eyes; they are a convergence of nutrition, convenience, and taste. Each bowl is a bold statement, a beautiful testament to the endless possibilities within the plant kingdom. This chapter is dedicated to these creations, inviting you to indulge in the art of bowl crafting with passion, purpose, and the spirit of the Vegan Vanguard.

The Philosophy of the Bowl

The bowl represents wholeness, a complete meal within its curved embrace. It's a philosophy of eating that combines various food groups to satisfy all the senses and nutritional needs. The Vegan Vanguard embraces this concept, creating bowls that are balanced in macronutrients, rich in micronutrients, and diverse in flavor profiles.

The Anatomy of a Perfect Bowl

Creating the perfect bowl is an art form. It starts with a base, typically grains or greens, followed by a variety of vegetables, a protein source, and a flavorful dressing or sauce. Toppings add texture and visual appeal, making each bowl a unique creation.

The Base: Grains and Greens

The foundation of any bowl is the base. Grains like quinoa, brown rice, or farro provide substance and are a source of complex carbohydrates. Greens like spinach, kale, or arugula offer a fresh contrast and are packed with vitamins.

The Veggies: Color and Crunch

Vegetables are the stars of the bowl, offering a spectrum of colors and a range of textures. Roasted sweet potatoes, steamed broccoli, sautéed mushrooms, or fresh avocado slices contribute to the bowl's nutritional density and visual appeal.

The Protein: Plant-Powered Muscle

Protein is essential, and in vegan bowls, it comes from sources like tofu, tempeh, lentils, or chickpeas. These ingredients not only add substance but also absorb the flavors of spices and dressings.

The Dressing: The Flavor Catalyst

A good dressing brings a bowl to life. Tahini lemon dressing, avocado cilantro lime, or a spicy peanut sauce can elevate the bowl from good to extraordinary.

The Toppings: The Final Flourish

Toppings like seeds, nuts, fresh herbs, or edible flowers add texture and a final flourish to the bowl, making it a true work of art.

Recipes for the Vanguard

Here are some recipes that embody the essence of the Vegan Vanguard's bold and beautiful bowls.

The Zen Garden Bowl

Ingredients:

1 cup cooked quinoa

1/2 cup edamame, shelled and cooked

1 carrot, julienned

1/2 cucumber, sliced

1/4 red cabbage, shredded

1/4 cup radishes, thinly sliced

1 avocado, sliced

Sesame seeds for garnish

Ginger miso dressing

Instructions:
1. Place quinoa at the bottom of the bowl as the base.
2. Arrange edamame, carrot, cucumber, red cabbage, radishes, and avocado in sections over the quinoa.
3. Drizzle with ginger miso dressing.
4. Garnish with sesame seeds.

The Mediterranean Sun Bowl
Ingredients:
1 cup cooked farro

1/2 cup hummus

1/2 cup cherry tomatoes, halved

1/2 cup cucumber, diced

1/4 cup of kalamata olives, pitted and halved

1/4 cup red onion, thinly sliced

1/4 cup artichoke hearts, quartered

A handful of arugula

Olive oil and lemon juice for dressing

Za'atar and fresh parsley for garnish

Instructions:
1. Spread farro as the base of the bowl.
2. Dollop hummus in the center.
3. Arrange tomatoes, cucumber, olives, red onion, and artichoke hearts around the hummus.
4. Tuck arugula into the sides of the bowl.

5. Pour lemon juice and olive oil over it.

6. Sprinkle za'atar and parsley on top.

Tips for Crafting Your Bowl

Balance Your Macros: Ensure each bowl has a good mix of carbohydrates, proteins, and fats.
Play with Textures: Combine crunchy, creamy, and chewy elements for an exciting eating experience.
Season Well: Don't forget to season each component of your bowl for maximum flavor.
Get Creative: Use what you have on hand and don't be afraid to try new combinations.

The bold and beautiful bowls of the Vegan Vanguard are more than just meals; they are a declaration of intent, a commitment to a lifestyle that is sustainable, ethical, and vibrant. Each bowl is a journey, a discovery of flavors, and a celebration of the abundance that a plant-based diet offers.

As you embark on your own bowl-making adventures, let your creativity run wild. Let each bowl you craft be a reflection of your personal journey, your connection to the earth, and your place in the Vegan Vanguard. For in the unity of ingredients within the confines of a bowl lies the unity of our cause: a healthier, kinder, and more beautiful world.

3:3 Savory Street Food: Recreating Favorite Street Eats Without Animal Products

Street food has the power to tell the story of a culture, to bring people together, and to offer a taste of home or a bite of adventure. It's the soul of many cities and the heartbeat of bustling markets. For the Vegan Vanguard, recreating these beloved flavors without animal products is not just a culinary challenge; it's a mission to prove that compassion and taste can go hand in hand. This chapter is a celebration of street food from around the globe, reimagined through a vegan lens.

The Art of Veganizing Street Food

The process of veganizing street food is an exercise in creativity and resourcefulness. It involves finding plant-based alternatives that can mimic the textures and flavors of traditional ingredients. Tofu, tempeh, jackfruit, and legumes stand in for meats; dairy-free cheeses and creams replace their animal-based counterparts; and a rainbow of vegetables, spices, and herbs bring dishes to life.

Recipes for the Urban Gourmet
Here are some recipes that capture the
essence of street food, each crafted with care
to ensure they are bursting with flavor and free
from animal products.

Vegan Tacos al Pastor
A Mexican classic, these tacos are traditionally
made with pork but here are reimagined with
marinated jackfruit for a similar texture and
taste.

Ingredients:
- 2 cans young green jackfruit in brine, drained
and shredded
- 2 tablespoons of finely chopped chipotle
chiles in adobo sauce

1 tablespoon achiote paste

1 tablespoon maple syrup

Juice of 1 lime

1 teaspoon cumin

1 teaspoon smoked paprika

Salt to taste

Corn tortillas

Pineapple slices, grilled

Red onion, finely chopped

Fresh cilantro, chopped

Instructions:
1. In a bowl, combine jackfruit, chipotle peppers, achiote paste, maple syrup, lime juice, cumin, smoked paprika, and salt. Give it at least half an hour to marinate.

2. Cook the jackfruit in a skillet over medium heat until it starts to caramelize, about 10 minutes.
3. Warm the tortillas on a skillet or directly over a flame.
4. Assemble the tacos by placing a spoonful of the jackfruit mixture on each tortilla, followed by a slice of grilled pineapple, red onion, and cilantro.

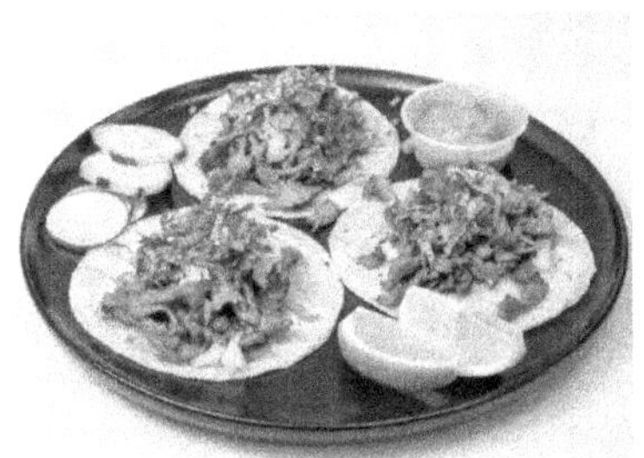

Tacos al Pastor

Vegan Banh Mi

This Vietnamese sandwich is a symphony of flavors and textures, featuring marinated tofu as the star.

Ingredients:
1 block firm tofu, pressed and sliced

1/4 cup soy sauce

1 tablespoon rice vinegar

1 tablespoon sesame oil

1 tablespoon maple syrup

1 garlic clove, minced

1 teaspoon grated ginger

Baguette or hoagie rolls, sliced open

Vegan mayonnaise

Pickled carrots and daikon radish

Cucumber slices

Jalapeño slices
Fresh cilantro

Instructions:
1. Whisk together soy sauce, rice vinegar, sesame oil, maple syrup, garlic, and ginger in a bowl. Marinate the tofu slices in this mixture for at least 1 hour.
2. Pan-fry the tofu until golden brown on both sides.
3. Spread vegan mayonnaise on the inside of the bread.
4. Layer the tofu, pickled vegetables, cucumber, jalapeño, and cilantro inside the bread.

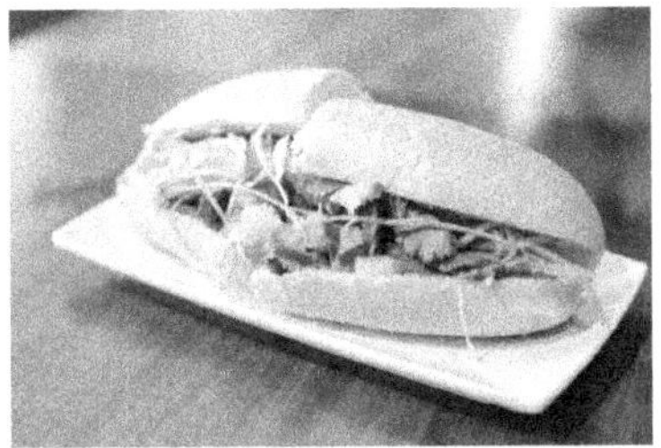

Beef Banh Mi Sandwich

Vegan Falafel Wrap

Falafel, the Middle Eastern gem, is naturally vegan and packed with flavor. Wrapped in a soft tortilla with fresh veggies and tahini sauce, it's a street food staple.

Ingredients:
2 cups of overnight-soaked and drained chickpeas
1 onion, chopped

2 garlic cloves

1/2 cup fresh parsley

1 teaspoon ground cumin

1 teaspoon ground coriander

Salt and pepper to taste

Vegetable oil for frying

Tortillas

Lettuce, shredded

Tomato, sliced

Tahini sauce

Instructions:
1. In a food processor, combine chickpeas, onion, garlic, parsley, cumin, coriander, salt, and pepper. Blend until well mixed, but do not puree.

2. Form the mixture into small patties or balls.
3. Heat oil in a deep pan and fry the falafel until golden and crispy.
4. Warm the tortillas, then fill with lettuce, tomato, and falafel.
5. Pour over some tahini sauce and firmly wrap.

Tips for Mastering Vegan Street Food

Experiment with Marinades: A good marinade can infuse vegan proteins with intense flavor.
Texture is Key: Play with cooking methods like grilling or frying to achieve the right texture.
Fresh Toppings: Use fresh herbs, pickles, and vegetables to add brightness and crunch to your dishes.

Street food is an expression of culture, a comfort for the soul, and a celebration of communal life. By bringing these flavors into the vegan fold, we honor the traditions of cuisines worldwide while forging a new path that is sustainable and ethical. These recipes are a call to action for all who believe in the power of plant-based eating, a rallying cry for the Vegan Vanguard to unite in the joy of cooking and the pleasure of sharing.

Let these savory street eats be a testament to the ingenuity and passion of vegan cooks everywhere. Let them inspire you to explore, to taste, and to create. For in every bite lies the potential for change, and in every dish, a story waiting to be told.

3:4 Sweet Indulgences: Irresistible Vegan Desserts

In the realm of veganism, desserts hold a special place. They are the grand finale to a meal, the sweet note that lingers on the palate, the indulgence that satisfies the soul. Crafting vegan desserts is an art form, a delicate balance of substituting traditional ingredients with plant-based alternatives without compromising on taste or texture. This chapter is a celebration of such sweet indulgences, a collection of irresistible vegan desserts that are sure to enchant and delight.

The Vanguard of Vegan Desserts
The Vegan Vanguard approaches desserts with reverence and innovation. They understand that desserts are more than just treats; they are expressions of culture, tradition, and creativity. With each recipe, they strive to honor the essence of classic sweets while infusing them with new life, ensuring that every creation is a testament to the joy and abundance of vegan living.

Decadent Chocolate Fudge Cake
A classic dessert reimagined, this chocolate fudge cake is rich, moist, and deeply chocolatey, proving that vegan desserts can be just as indulgent as their non-vegan counterparts.

Ingredients:
2 cups all-purpose flour

1 1/2 cups of organic sugar

3/4 cup cocoa powder

2 teaspoons baking powder

1 1/2 teaspoons baking soda

1 teaspoon salt

1 teaspoon instant coffee powder (optional)

1 cup non-dairy milk

1/2 cup vegetable oil

2 teaspoons vanilla extract

1 cup boiling water

Vegan chocolate frosting

Instructions:
1. Preheat your oven to 350°F (175°C). Get a 9 inch cake pan and grease it
2. In a large bowl, whisk together flour, sugar, cocoa, baking powder, baking soda, salt, and coffee powder.
3. Add non-dairy milk, vegetable oil, and vanilla extract. Mix until well combined.
4. Stir in boiling water until the batter is smooth (it will be thin).
5. Evenly divide the batter between the prepared pans.
6. Bake for about 30 to 35 minutes, or better still, until a toothpick inserted into the center comes out clean and smoothly.
7. Let cool completely before frosting with vegan chocolate frosting.

Luscious Lemon Tart
Bright, tangy, and utterly refreshing, this lemon tart has a silky-smooth filling encased in a buttery crust, perfect for those who crave a zestier dessert.

Ingredients:
For the crust:

1 1/4 cups all-purpose flour

1/4 cup organic sugar

1/4 teaspoon salt

1/2 cup vegan butter, cold and cubed

2 tablespoons ice water

For the filling:
1 cup organic sugar

2 tablespoons all-purpose flour

3/4 cup fresh lemon juice

Zest of 2 lemons

1/2 cup non-dairy milk

4 tablespoons cornstarch

Pinch of turmeric for color (optional)

Instructions:
1. For the crust, pulse flour, sugar, and salt in a
food processor. Add vegan butter and pulse

until crumbly. Add ice water and pulse until a dough forms.

2. Press the dough into a tart pan and bake at 350°F (175°C) for 15 minutes.

3. For the filling, whisk together sugar, flour, lemon juice, lemon zest, non-dairy milk, cornstarch, and turmeric in a saucepan over medium heat.

4. Cook, stirring constantly, until the mixture thickens. Pour into the baked crust.

5. Chill in the refrigerator for at least 2 hours before serving.

Heavenly Raspberry Sorbet

This raspberry sorbet is a palate cleanser, a dessert that is both light and intensely flavorful, capturing the essence of fresh raspberries in every spoonful.

Ingredients:

4 cups fresh raspberries

3/4 cup organic sugar

1 cup water

Juice of 1 lemon

Instructions:
1. In a saucepan, combine sugar and water. Heat until the sugar dissolves.
2. Blend raspberries and lemon juice in a blender until smooth.
3. Strain the raspberry mixture through a fine-mesh sieve to remove seeds.
4. Stir the raspberry puree into the sugar syrup.
5. Chill the mixture in the refrigerator, then churn in an ice cream maker according to the manufacturer's instructions.

Tips for Crafting Vegan Desserts

Quality Ingredients: Use the best quality ingredients for the best results. Organic fruits, high-quality cocoa, and pure extracts make a difference.

Patience is Key: Allow desserts to cool and set properly before serving. This patience pays off in texture and taste.

Presentation Matters: Take time to present your desserts beautifully. A sprig of mint, a dusting of powdered sugar, or a drizzle of sauce can elevate the visual appeal.

Vegan desserts are a celebration, a sweet indulgence that can be enjoyed without compromise. They are a testament to the creativity and passion of those who choose to live a vegan lifestyle. Each recipe in this collection is crafted with care, ensuring that every dessert is not just a treat for the taste buds but also a reflection of the Vegan Vanguard's commitment to compassion and excellence.

Let these sweet indulgences be a source of joy and inspiration. Let them remind you that veganism is not about restriction but about discovery, innovation, and the sheer pleasure of good food. For in the world of vegan desserts, there are no limits—only possibilities waiting to be explored and enjoyed.

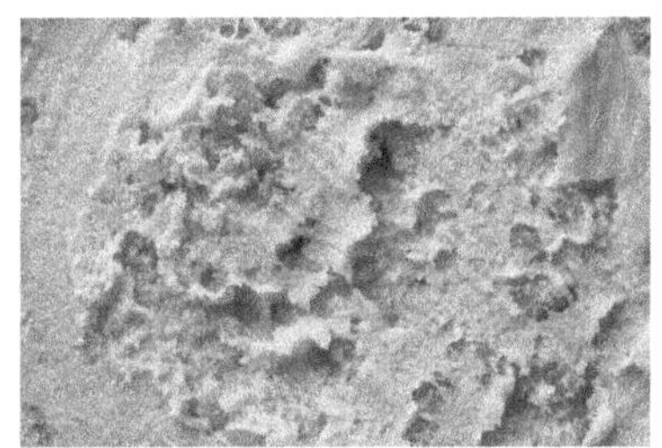

Raspberry Sorbet ice cream

CHAPTER FOUR

Sustainable Strategies: Forging a Future with Intention and Integrity

In the quest for a sustainable future, the choices we make today are the seeds of tomorrow's world. The Vegan Vanguard stands at the forefront of this movement, championing a lifestyle that is not only ethical and compassionate but also environmentally conscious. This chapter delves into the myriad of strategies that can be employed to create a sustainable lifestyle, each one interwoven with the passion and purpose that define the Vegan Vanguard.

The Pillars of Sustainability

Sustainability is built upon three fundamental pillars: environmental protection, social equity, and economic viability. Each pillar is crucial, and together, they form a framework for a world that can thrive for generations to come.

Environmental Protection: The Earth as Our Sanctuary

The first pillar, environmental protection, calls for a profound respect for our natural world. It is a commitment to preserving biodiversity, conserving resources, and minimizing waste. The Vegan Vanguard embraces this through practices such as:

Plant-Based Diet: Recognizing that a diet centered around plant-based foods significantly reduces one's carbon footprint and conserves water.

Zero-Waste Living: Striving to eliminate waste by reducing, reusing, and recycling, and by choosing products with minimal packaging.

Conservation Efforts: Engaging in activities that protect natural habitats, such as supporting reforestation projects or participating in clean-up drives.

Social Equity: The Heart of Humanity

The second pillar, social equity, is about ensuring fair treatment, access, and advancement for all people. It is about building communities that are inclusive, diverse, and just. The Vegan Vanguard advocates for social equity by:

Community Support: Working with local communities to support food security initiatives, such as community gardens or plant-based food banks.
Education and Outreach: Sharing knowledge about the benefits of a vegan lifestyle and providing resources for those interested in making the transition.
Fair Trade: Choosing products that are certified fair trade, ensuring that producers in developing countries are paid a fair wage.

Economic Viability: Prosperity with Purpose
The third pillar, economic viability, involves creating systems that promote economic prosperity while respecting ecological and social boundaries. The Vegan Vanguard contributes to this by:

Supporting Sustainable Businesses:
Patronizing companies that have sustainable practices and ethical business models.
Green Investments: Investing in green technologies and industries that are leading the way in sustainability.
Mindful Consumption: Being conscious consumers, purchasing only what is needed,

and opting for products that have a long lifespan.

Strategies for Sustainable Living

Living sustainably is about making intentional choices. Here are some strategies that anyone can adopt to live in harmony with our planet:

Reduce Energy Consumption: Switch to energy-efficient appliances, use LED lighting, and unplug electronics when not in use.

Water conservation: Replace low-flow fixtures, take shorter showers, and address leaks.

Choose Sustainable Transportation: Walk, bike, use public transportation, or carpool whenever possible.

Eat Locally and Seasonally: Support local farmers and reduce the carbon footprint associated with transporting food long distances.

Minimize Food Waste: Plan meals, store food properly, and compost organic waste.

Green Your Home: Use non-toxic cleaning products, plant a garden, and use natural materials in home decor.

The Role of Technology in Sustainability
Technology plays a pivotal role in advancing sustainability. Innovations such as renewable energy, sustainable agriculture, and water purification systems are changing the way we live. The Vegan Vanguard embraces technology that:

Promotes Renewable Energy: Solar panels, wind turbines, and other renewable energy sources are key to reducing reliance on fossil fuels.

Advanced Sustainable Agriculture: Techniques like vertical farming, hydroponics, and aquaponics are making it possible to grow food in more sustainable ways.

Improves Resource Management: Smart technologies that optimize the use of resources can lead to significant reductions in waste and consumption.

The Vegan Vanguard's Commitment
The Vegan Vanguard's commitment to sustainability is unwavering. It is a lifestyle choice that encompasses every aspect of living, from the food on the plate to the clothes on one's back. It is a call to action for mindful living, for making decisions that align with the

values of compassion, respect, and stewardship.

Sustainability is not a destination but a journey, one that requires constant learning, adapting, and growing. There will be difficulties along the way, but there will also be great benefits. As members of the Vegan Vanguard, we have the opportunity to lead by example, to show the world that it is possible to live in a way that honors all forms of life and preserves the beauty and bounty of our planet.

Let us move forward with intention and integrity, with the knowledge that our actions today shape the world of tomorrow. Let us be the change we wish to see, and let our legacy be one of a sustainable, just, and thriving planet for all.

4:1 Eco-Conscious Cooking: Reducing Food Waste and Minimizing Environmental Impact

In the heart of every eco-conscious kitchen, there lies a commitment to sustainability that goes beyond the plate. It's a philosophy that intertwines the love for cooking with the responsibility we hold towards our planet. Eco-conscious cooking is about making deliberate choices that reduce food waste and minimize environmental impact, ensuring that our culinary practices contribute to a healthier world.

The Essence of Eco-Conscious Cooking

Eco-conscious cooking starts with an awareness of the resources we use and the waste we produce. It's a holistic approach that considers the lifecycle of food, from farm to fork to compost. This method of cooking is a powerful tool in the fight against climate change, as it seeks to lower greenhouse gas emissions and conserve biodiversity.

Strategies for Sustainable Cooking

Here are some strategies that embody the principles of eco-conscious cooking, each designed to make a positive impact on the environment:

Mindful Meal Planning: Plan your meals to use ingredients efficiently, purchasing only what you need and using leftovers creatively to prevent waste.

Seasonal and Local Eating: Choose ingredients that are in season and locally sourced to reduce the carbon footprint associated with transportation and storage.

Conservation Cooking Techniques: Opt for energy-efficient cooking methods like steaming, pressure cooking, or using a slow cooker.

Composting: Turn food scraps into nutrient-rich compost to enrich the soil and reduce methane emissions from landfills.

Packaging Awareness: Reduce reliance on single-use plastics by choosing bulk items, bringing reusable bags, and selecting products with minimal packaging.

Recipes for the Earth-Friendly Foodie

The following recipes are crafted with the earth in mind, each one a celebration of flavors that respects our environment.

Sustainable Stir-Fry
A versatile dish that allows you to use a variety of seasonal vegetables, reducing waste and supporting local produce.

Ingredients:
2 cups of mixed seasonal vegetables (e.g., bell peppers, zucchini, carrots)

1 cup of tofu, cubed

2 tablespoons of soy sauce

1 tablespoon of sesame oil

1 garlic clove, minced

1 teaspoon of grated ginger

Cooked rice or noodles, for serving

Instructions:

1. In a pan that is over medium heat, heat the
sesame oil. Add tofu and cook until golden
brown. Remove and set aside.
2. In the same pan, add garlic and ginger,
sautéing until fragrant.
3. Add the mixed vegetables and stir-fry until
just tender.
4. Return the tofu to the pan, pour in soy
sauce, and toss everything together.
5. Serve over rice or noodles.

Zero-Waste Vegetable Broth

A flavorful broth made from vegetable scraps
that would otherwise be discarded.

Ingredients:
vegetable leftovers, such as celery leaves,
carrot tops, and onion peels

1 bay leaf

1 teaspoon of whole peppercorns

Salt to taste

Water

Instructions:
1. Collect and clean vegetable scraps, ensuring they are free from dirt.
2. Place the scraps in a large pot and fill with water until covered.
3. Add bay leaf, peppercorns, and salt.
4. After bringing to a boil, lower the heat, and simmer for one hour.
5. Strain the broth and use it as a base for soups, stews, or cooking grains.

Tips for Eco-Conscious Cooking

Embrace Imperfection: Use fruits and vegetables that are slightly bruised or misshapen instead of discarding them.
Energy Efficiency: Cook multiple dishes in the oven simultaneously or use residual heat to finish cooking.
Water Wisdom: Use minimal water for cooking and repurpose water used for washing vegetables to water plants.
Preservation: Learn preservation techniques like canning, drying, or pickling to extend the life of seasonal produce.

The Impact of Eco-Conscious Cooking

By adopting eco-conscious cooking practices, we can make a significant impact on our environment. We can reduce our carbon footprint, support sustainable agriculture, and contribute to a reduction in global food waste. It's a way of cooking that not only nourishes our bodies but also protects our planet.

Eco-conscious cooking is an act of love—love for food, love for people, and love for the earth. It's a journey that begins in the kitchen and extends to the global community, a path that the Vegan Vanguard walks with pride and purpose. Let us cook with intention, eat with gratitude, and live with the knowledge that our choices have the power to shape a sustainable future.

Let this chapter serve as a guide and an inspiration for all who wish to embrace eco-conscious cooking. Let it be a reminder that every meal is an opportunity to make a difference, and every dish a step towards a more sustainable world.

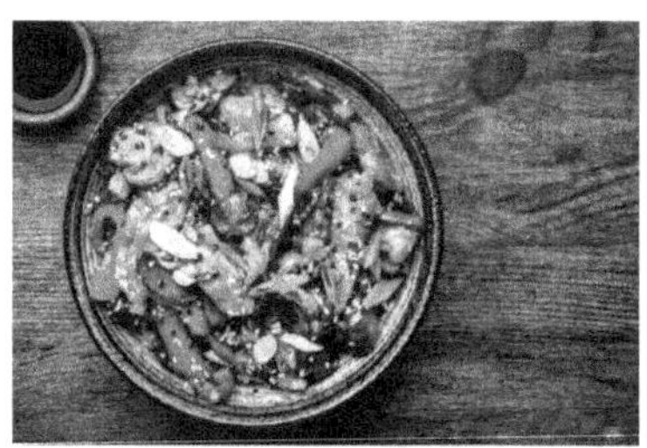

Stir fry chicken with paprika, mushrooms and chives.

4:2 Seasonal Eating: Celebrating the Bounty of Each Season

In the dance of the seasons, nature offers a symphony of flavors, colors, and textures. Seasonal eating is the act of harmonizing our diets with the rhythm of nature, selecting fruits and vegetables that are naturally at their peak. It's a practice as old as time, rooted in the wisdom of our ancestors who followed the cycles of the earth to nourish themselves. Today, the Vegan Vanguard rekindles this tradition with a modern twist, embracing the bounty of each season with a passion for sustainability and a commitment to the health of our planet.

The Spring Awakening

As winter's chill gives way to the gentle warmth of spring, the earth awakens with a burst of life. Tender greens, sweet peas, and bright berries make their debut, signaling a time of renewal and growth. Spring's bounty is a reminder of the earth's resilience, offering foods that cleanse and rejuvenate the body after the hearty fare of colder months.

Recipes for Rejuvenation

Spring Pea and Mint Soup: A vibrant blend of fresh peas, aromatic mint, and rich vegetable broth, pureed to silky perfection.
Strawberry Spinach Salad: A refreshing mix of sweet strawberries, tender spinach, and crunchy almonds, dressed in a zesty balsamic vinaigrette.

The Summer's Abundance
Summer arrives with a flourish, draping the landscape in a tapestry of lushness. Juicy tomatoes, crisp cucumbers, and succulent stone fruits are just a few of the season's treasures. Meals become a celebration of color and flavor, with an emphasis on freshness and simplicity.

Recipes for Celebration

Heirloom Tomato Gazpacho: A cold soup that captures the essence of ripe tomatoes, enhanced with the flavors of fresh herbs and a hint of garlic.
Peach and Basil Sorbet: A sweet and aromatic dessert that pairs the lusciousness of peaches with the subtle spice of basil.

The Autumn Harvest

Autumn heralds a time of abundance, a season to gather and give thanks. Root vegetables, hearty squashes, and crisp apples are the stars of the show, offering warmth and sustenance as the air turns cool. This is a time for comforting dishes that satisfy the soul and celebrate the harvest.

Recipes for Comfort

Roasted Butternut Squash Soup: A creamy soup that showcases the natural sweetness of squash, complemented by the depth of roasted garlic and the warmth of ginger.
Apple Cinnamon Crumble: A classic dessert with tender apples and a crunchy topping, redolent with the spices of cinnamon and nutmeg.

The Winter

Winter wraps the world in a blanket of quietude, a season for introspection and rest. Citrus fruits burst onto the scene, offering a splash of sunshine amid the gray. Root vegetables and dark leafy greens continue to provide nourishment, grounding us through the coldest months.

Recipes for Nourishment

Citrus and Fennel Salad: A crisp and refreshing salad that combines the tang of citrus with the anise-like flavor of fennel, dressed in a light citrus vinaigrette.
Kale and White Bean Stew: A hearty and warming stew that pairs the robustness of kale with the creaminess of white beans, flavored with rosemary and thyme.

The Vanguard's Approach to Seasonal Eating

The Vegan Vanguard approaches seasonal eating with mindfulness and intention. They understand that what we eat not only affects our health but also the health of our planet. By choosing seasonal produce, they support local farmers, reduce the carbon footprint associated with transportation, and enjoy foods that are at their nutritional peak.

Tips for Seasonal Eating

Visit Local Farmers' Markets: Connect with local growers and discover the variety of produce that each season brings.
Preserve the Harvest: Learn techniques like canning, freezing, or fermenting to enjoy seasonal flavors all year round.
Get Creative in the Kitchen: Use seasonal produce as an inspiration for new dishes, experimenting with flavors and cooking methods.

Seasonal eating is a journey through the year, a way to live in harmony with the earth's cycles. It's an opportunity to reconnect with the sources of our food, to appreciate the natural ebb and flow of growth and dormancy. The Vegan Vanguard embraces this cycle with enthusiasm, recognizing that each season brings its own unique gifts.

Let us celebrate the bounty of each season with gratitude and joy. Let us cook with the knowledge that our choices can lead to a more sustainable and compassionate world. For in the simple act of eating seasonally, we find a profound connection to the earth and a path to a better future.

4:3 Zero-Waste Kitchen Hacks: Practical Tips for a Greener Kitchen

In the heart of the home, the kitchen is a place of creation and nourishment. Yet, it is also a place where waste can easily accumulate. Adopting a zero-waste approach in the kitchen is not only an act of environmental stewardship but also a step towards a more mindful and sustainable lifestyle. This chapter is dedicated to practical tips and hacks that can transform your kitchen into a greener space, aligning with the Vegan Vanguard's ethos of passion, purpose, and the spirit of positive change.

Understanding Zero-Waste

The zero-waste movement is about rethinking our relationship with materials and resources, aiming to reduce what we send to landfills and incinerators to the absolute minimum. It's about finding value in what we already have and making the most of it. In the kitchen, this translates to a series of practices that minimize food waste and reduce the use of disposable items.

Comprehensive Composting

One of the cornerstones of a zero-waste kitchen is composting. By turning organic waste into nutrient-rich compost, you not only reduce methane emissions from landfills but also contribute to soil health. Arrange eggshells, coffee grounds, and leftover fruit and vegetable scraps in a compost bin in your kitchen. If you don't have a garden, find out about local composting initiatives.

Mindful Shopping

Shopping with a zero-waste mindset is crucial. Bring reusable bags and containers to the grocery store to avoid unnecessary packaging. Shop in bulk when possible, and choose products with minimal or recyclable packaging. Prioritize fresh produce over processed foods, and buy only what you need to avoid spoilage.

Efficient Food Storage

Proper food storage is key to preventing waste. Invest in reusable containers, beeswax wraps, and silicone lids to keep food fresh longer. Learn the best ways to store different types of produce, and make sure to use the oldest items first. Keep your fridge organized so you can see everything at a glance, reducing the chance of forgotten items spoiling.

Creative Cooking

Get creative in the kitchen by using every part of the food. Vegetable peels, stems, and leaves can be used to make stocks and broths. Overripe fruits work well in smoothies or baked goods. Stale bread can become croutons or breadcrumbs. Challenge yourself to find new uses for what might otherwise be thrown away.

DIY Cleaning Products

Reduce the need for single-use plastic bottles by making your own cleaning products. Simple ingredients like vinegar, baking soda, and lemon can be used to create effective and natural cleaners. Keep them in spray bottles or reusable glass jars.

Energy and Water Efficiency

Be conscious of your energy and water use. Cook with lids on to reduce cooking times, and use the right size burner for your pots and pans. Fill the sink with water for washing dishes rather than letting the tap run. If you want to lower water flow without compromising pressure, install aerators on your faucets.

Sustainable Utensils and Cookware

Choose durable and sustainably made utensils and cookware. Opt for items made from stainless steel, cast iron, or bamboo, which can last for years and are often recyclable at the end of their life. Avoid single-use items like plastic utensils and paper plates.

Growing Your Own

Grow and produce your own veggies and herbs, if you have the space.. Even a small windowsill garden can provide fresh flavors for your cooking and reduce the need for store-bought produce.

Educating and Sharing

Share your zero-waste journey with friends and family. Educate others on the importance of reducing waste and how they can implement these practices in their own homes. The more people join the movement, the greater the impact.

The Vegan Vanguard's Vision

The Vegan Vanguard envisions a world where our daily actions are in harmony with the environment. A zero-waste kitchen is a reflection of this vision, a place where every resource is valued, and nothing is taken for granted. It's a testament to the belief that small changes can lead to significant impacts.

Transforming your kitchen into a zero-waste space is a journey of intention and commitment. It's about making choices that align with a deeper understanding of our impact on the planet. The tips provided in this chapter are stepping stones towards a greener kitchen, each one an action that supports the Vegan Vanguard's mission for a sustainable future.

Let these hacks inspire you to rethink, repurpose, and rejuvenate your approach to cooking and kitchen management. Embrace the challenge with passion, fulfill it with purpose, and let the spirit of the Vegan Vanguard guide you towards a zero-waste life.

4:4 Grow Your Own: Starting a Small Herb or Vegetable Garden

In the embrace of nature, there is a profound sense of connection and accomplishment that comes from cultivating your own food. Starting a small herb or vegetable garden is a journey back to the roots of sustenance, an act that ties us to the cycles of life and growth. For the Vegan Vanguard, this practice is more than a hobby; it's a statement of self-reliance, sustainability, and a step towards a more conscious way of living.

The Groundwork of Gardening

Gardening begins with understanding the soil beneath our feet. It's about creating a nurturing environment where plants can flourish. Begin by assessing the quality of your soil. Is it sandy, clay-heavy, or loamy? The texture of your soil will determine how well it retains water and nutrients. Enriching your soil with compost or organic matter can improve its structure and fertility, creating a hospitable bed for your plants to grow.

Choosing Your Crops

Selecting what to grow is a delightful dilemma. Start with herbs and vegetables that you enjoy eating and that are known to thrive in your climate. Herbs like basil, cilantro, and mint are excellent for beginners, as they grow quickly and don't require much space. Vegetables such as tomatoes, lettuce, and radishes are also good starter plants, offering quick gratification and a variety of uses in the kitchen.

Sowing Seeds of Success

Planting your garden is a dance with timing and technique. Some plants prefer the cool days of early spring, while others need the warmth of summer to prosper. Research the best time to sow each type of seed in your region. When planting, consider the spacing requirements for each plant, allowing them room to grow without competition. Water your seeds gently and keep the soil moist to encourage germination.

Tending to Your Garden

As your plants sprout and stretch towards the sun, they will require care and attention. Regular watering is essential, but be mindful not to overwater, as this can lead to root rot.

Weeding is also crucial, as weeds can steal nutrients and sunlight from your plants. As your vegetables and herbs mature, they may need support structures like stakes or trellises to help them reach their full potential.

Harvesting with Heart

The harvest is a time of celebration, a moment to reap the rewards of your labor. Harvest your herbs and vegetables when they are at their peak of ripeness for the best flavor. Use scissors or pruners to cut herbs, encouraging further growth. For vegetables, be gentle to avoid damaging the plant or its roots. Remember, the more you harvest, the more your plants will produce.

From Garden to Table

Bringing your homegrown produce into the kitchen is an act of joy. Fresh herbs can transform a simple dish into something extraordinary. Vegetables from your garden carry the flavors of the earth and the care you've invested in them. Create meals that showcase the freshness of your harvest, and share them with friends and family to spread the love of homegrown food.

Sustainable Practices

In line with the Vegan Vanguard's commitment to sustainability, consider implementing practices that reduce waste and promote ecological balance. Collect rainwater for irrigation, use natural pest deterrents like companion planting, and save seeds from your plants for the next growing season.

Expanding Your Green Thumb

As you gain confidence and experience, you may wish to expand your garden. Experiment with new varieties of herbs and vegetables, or try your hand at fruit-bearing plants. Each new plant brings its own set of challenges and rewards, adding depth and diversity to your gardening experience.

The Vegan Vanguard's Vision

For the Vegan Vanguard, gardening is a reflection of their values, a testament to the belief that we can live in harmony with the earth and take control of our food sources. It's a step towards a future where communities are self-sustaining and where the bond between human and nature is revered.

Starting a small herb or vegetable garden is a journey of discovery, a path that leads to a deeper understanding of nature's cycles and our place within them. It's an endeavor that requires patience, care, and a willingness to learn. But the rewards are immeasurable, not just in the food that graces our tables, but in the knowledge that we are contributing to a more sustainable and compassionate world.

Let this guide be the seed from which your garden grows. Let it inspire you to take up the trowel and plant with purpose, passion, and the spirit of the Vegan Vanguard. For in every seed lies the potential for growth, and in every garden, a promise for the future.

CHAPTER FIVE

Vanguard for Life: Embodying the Essence of Conscious Living

The term 'vanguard' evokes images of pioneers, leaders, and trailblazers. It is about being at the forefront of movements, ideas, and changes that shape the world. For those who identify with the Vegan Vanguard, it is a lifelong commitment to living consciously, compassionately, and sustainably. This chapter is a deep dive into what it means to be a vanguard for life, exploring the principles that guide this journey and the practices that define it.

Living with Intention

To be a vanguard for life is to live with intention. It is to make choices that are deliberate and thoughtful, with an awareness of the impact they have on oneself, others, and the planet. It is about aligning actions with values, ensuring that every step taken is a step towards a better future.

Compassion as a Guiding Principle

At the heart of the Vegan Vanguard's philosophy is compassion. Compassion for animals, leading to a plant-based diet free from animal products; compassion for fellow humans, fostering a culture of kindness and equity; and compassion for the earth, promoting actions that safeguard and maintain the environment.

Sustainability as a Way of Life

Sustainability is a way of life, not just a trendy term. It involves making choices that meet present needs without compromising the ability of future generations to meet theirs. From reducing waste to conserving resources, every aspect of daily life is an opportunity to contribute to a more sustainable world.

Advocacy and Activism

Being part of the vanguard means being an advocate and an activist. It is about using one's voice to speak up for those who cannot, whether they be animals, marginalized communities, or the environment. It is about taking action, whether through peaceful protests, educational outreach, or political engagement.

Health and Wellbeing
The Vegan Vanguard places a high value on health and wellbeing, recognizing that personal health is deeply connected to the health of the planet. A balanced, plant-based diet, regular exercise, and mindfulness practices are all integral to maintaining physical and mental wellbeing.

Continuous Learning
The journey of the vanguard is one of continuous learning. It is about staying informed, being open to new ideas, and adapting to change. It is about seeking knowledge, whether through books, documentaries, or conversations, and using that knowledge to make informed decisions.

Community and Connection
No vanguard stands alone. Community and connection are vital, providing support, inspiration, and a sense of belonging. Building relationships with like-minded individuals,

participating in community events, and collaborating on projects are all ways to strengthen the movement and foster unity.

Creativity and Innovation

The vanguard's vitality is derived from creativity and innovation. They are about finding new solutions to old problems, thinking outside the box, and being unafraid to try something different. Whether it's developing new vegan recipes, designing sustainable products, or creating art that inspires change, creativity is a powerful tool for progress.

Resilience and Perseverance

The path of the vanguard is not always easy. It requires resilience and perseverance in the face of challenges and setbacks. It is about staying true to one's convictions, even when it is difficult, and continuing to push forward towards the vision of a better world.

The Spirit of the Vanguard

The spirit of the Vanguard is one of hope, determination, and unwavering commitment. It is a spirit that burns brightly, driving the movement forward and illuminating the path for others to follow. It is a spirit that is contagious, inspiring others to join the cause and become vanguards in their own right.

To be a vanguard for life is a profound and noble pursuit. It is a commitment that extends beyond diet or lifestyle; it is a commitment to being an agent of change in every aspect of life. It is about embodying the principles of conscious living, day in and day out, with passion, purpose, and the spirit of the Vegan Vanguard.

Let this chapter serve as a manifesto for all who aspire to be vanguards for life. Let it be a call to action, a source of inspiration, and a reminder that each of us has the power to make a difference. For in the end, the vanguard is not just a group of individuals; it is a movement, a collective force that has the potential to transform the world.

5:1 Mindful Eating Practices: Cultivating Awareness Around Food Choices

In the journey towards a more conscious lifestyle, the way we approach our meals plays a pivotal role. Mindful eating is not merely a practice but a philosophy that intertwines the act of nourishment with presence and awareness. It's about engaging all our senses to experience the full spectrum of our food's journey, from its origins to its effects on our bodies and minds. For the Vegan Vanguard, mindful eating is a fundamental aspect of their ethos, reflecting a deep commitment to making food choices that are ethical, sustainable, and health-promoting.

The Essence of Mindfulness

Mindfulness is the quality of being fully present and engaged in the moment, aware of our thoughts, feelings, bodily sensations, and surrounding environment. When applied to eating, mindfulness transforms the act into a meditative experience, encouraging a deeper connection with the food we consume.

Cultivating Mindful Eating Habits

To cultivate mindful eating, one must begin with intention. It starts before a meal is even prepared, with the selection of ingredients. Choosing foods that are ethically sourced, organically grown, and locally produced whenever possible is a conscious decision that supports not only personal health but also the health of the planet.

Creating a Mindful Space

The environment in which we eat can significantly influence our level of mindfulness. Creating a calm and comfortable dining space, free from distractions like television or smartphones, allows us to focus on the act of eating. A clean and organized setting invites us to appreciate the colors, textures, and aromas of our food, setting the stage for a mindful meal.

Engaging the Senses

Mindful eating involves engaging all five senses. We observe the visual appeal of our food, we savor its aroma, we listen to the sounds of cooking or the crunch of fresh produce, we delight in the texture as we chew, and we taste every nuanced flavor. This sensory engagement slows down the eating process, allowing us to recognize when we are full and to appreciate the nourishment our food provides.

Acknowledging the Journey of Food
Each bite we take is the culmination of a vast journey. Mindful eating practices involve acknowledging the journey our food has taken to reach our plates—the soil it grew in, the hands that harvested it, the journey it traveled, and the transformation it underwent. This acknowledgment fosters gratitude and a sense of connection to the world around us.

Listening to the Body
Mindful eating also means listening to our bodies' signals. It's about eating when we're truly hungry and stopping when we're satisfied. It encourages us to notice how different foods affect our energy, mood, and overall well-being, guiding us to make choices that serve us best.

Mindful Preparation and Cooking

The act of preparing and cooking food is also an opportunity for mindfulness. It's a time to be fully engaged in the process, to experiment with flavors and techniques, and to infuse our meals with care and intention. Cooking becomes a joyful and creative endeavor, rather than a chore or routine.

The Role of Mindful Eating in the Vegan Vanguard

For the Vegan Vanguard, mindful eating is a reflection of their values. It is a practice that embodies their commitment to living with purpose and passion. It's a way to honor the lives of all beings, to tread lightly on the earth, and to nourish themselves in a way that is aligned with their vision for a better world.

Mindful Eating as a Path to Transformation

Mindful eating has the power to transform our relationship with food. It turns each meal into an opportunity for growth, learning, and connection. It's a practice that can lead to healthier eating habits, a greater appreciation for the abundance of the earth, and a deeper understanding of the impact of our food choices.

Mindful eating is more than a technique; it's a way of life. It's an integral part of the Vegan Vanguard's journey, a path that leads to greater awareness, compassion, and sustainability. By embracing mindful eating practices, we open ourselves to a more fulfilling and conscious way of living, one that honors our bodies, our planet, and all its inhabitants.

Let this exploration of mindful eating inspire you to approach your meals with a new perspective. Let it encourage you to slow down, to savor, and to choose with care. For in the act of eating mindfully, we find not only nourishment for our bodies but also nourishment for our souls.

5:2 Vegan on the Go: Quick and Satisfying Meals for Busy Days

In the hustle and bustle of modern life, finding time for a nutritious meal can often be a challenge, especially for those committed to a vegan lifestyle. The key to maintaining this commitment without compromising on taste or nutrition lies in mastering the art of 'Vegan on the Go'—quick, satisfying meals that cater to a busy schedule. This chapter is dedicated to the Vegan Vanguard, offering a collection of recipes and tips designed to fuel your day with plant-based goodness, all while keeping pace with your active life.

The Philosophy of 'Vegan on the Go'
The philosophy behind 'Vegan on the Go' is simple: quick preparation, nutritional balance, and undeniable flavor. It's about having a repertoire of meals that can be assembled in minutes, providing the energy and sustenance needed to power through the day. These meals are portable, convenient, and tailored to fit into a compact, fast-paced lifestyle.

Building a 'Vegan on the Go' Pantry

A well-stocked pantry is the foundation of quick and easy vegan meals. Essentials include canned beans, whole grain wraps, pre-cooked grains, nuts, seeds, and a variety of spices and condiments. With these staples on hand, you're always ready to whip up a meal in no time.

Recipes for the Rapid Vegan

Here are some recipes that embody the essence of 'Vegan on the Go', each one crafted to be prepared swiftly, enjoyed heartily, and packed with nutrition.

Chickpea Salad Wrap

A refreshing and protein-packed wrap that's as easy to make as it is delicious.

Ingredients:

1 can chickpeas, drained and rinsed

1/4 cup vegan mayonnaise

1 tablespoon Dijon mustard

1/2 red onion, finely chopped

1 celery stalk, finely chopped

1/4 cup pickles, chopped

Salt and pepper to taste

Whole grain wraps

Lettuce leaves

Instructions:
1. Mash the chickpeas in a bowl using a fork or potato masher.
2. Stir in vegan mayonnaise, Dijon mustard, red onion, celery, and pickles. Season with salt and pepper.
3. Lay a whole grain wrap on a flat surface, place a lettuce leaf in the center, and spoon the chickpea mixture onto the lettuce.
4. Roll up the wrap tightly, cut in half, and it's ready to go.

Overnight Oats Jar
A no-cook, make-ahead breakfast that's perfect for those mornings when you're short on time.

Ingredients:
1/2 cup rolled oats

1 tablespoon chia seeds

1 cup almond milk

1 tablespoon maple syrup

1/2 teaspoon vanilla extract

Toppings: fresh fruits, nuts, seeds

Instructions:
1. In a jar, combine rolled oats, chia seeds, almond milk, maple syrup, and vanilla extract.
2. Stir well, seal the jar, and refrigerate overnight.
3. In the morning, add your favorite toppings, and enjoy straight from the jar.

Quick Quinoa Bowl
A versatile and hearty bowl that can be customized with whatever veggies and toppings you have on hand.

Ingredients:
1 cup cooked quinoa

1/2 cup of rinsed and drained black beans

1/2 avocado, sliced

1/2 cup cherry tomatoes, halved

1/4 cup corn kernels

1/4 cup red bell pepper, diced

2 tablespoons salsa

A squeeze of lime juice

Cilantro for garnish

Instructions:
1. In a bowl, layer the cooked quinoa, black beans, avocado, cherry tomatoes, corn, and red bell pepper.
2. Top with salsa, a squeeze of lime juice, and garnish with cilantro.
3. Mix everything together and enjoy.

Tips for 'Vegan on the Go' Success

Meal Prep: Dedicate time to meal prep. Cook grains and legumes in bulk and chop veggies ahead of time.
Portable Containers: Invest in quality, leak-proof containers that make transportation easy and mess-free.

Snack Smart: Keep a stash of portable vegan snacks like fruit, nuts, or energy bars for when hunger strikes.

Maintain Hydration: Carry a reusable water bottle to ensure you stay hydrated throughout the day.

The Vegan Vanguard's Commitment

For the Vegan Vanguard, 'Vegan on the Go' is more than just a convenience; it's a commitment to maintaining their plant-based principles, even in the midst of a hectic schedule. It's about making conscious food choices that reflect their dedication to health, compassion, and sustainability.

'Vegan on the Go' is a testament to the fact that a busy lifestyle doesn't have to mean compromised values or nutrition. With a bit of planning and creativity, you can enjoy quick, satisfying vegan meals that align with the Vegan Vanguard's vision of a vibrant, healthful life. Let these recipes and tips inspire you to embrace the convenience of 'Vegan on the Go', infusing your days with passion, purpose, and the spirit of the vegan vanguard.

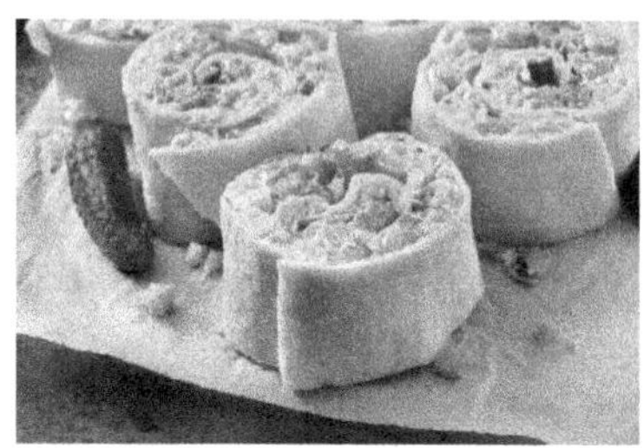

Creamy Chickpea Salad Tortilla Wraps

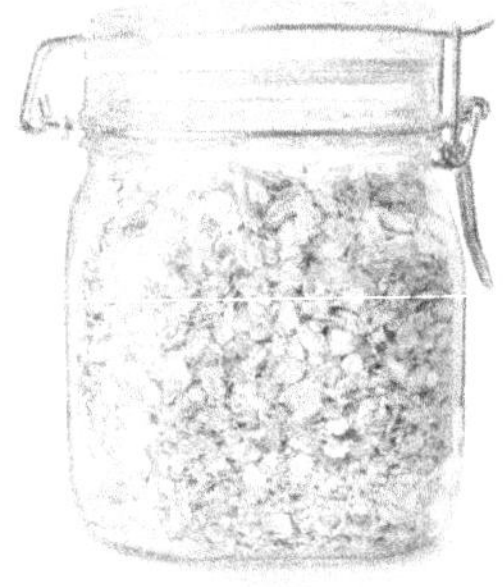

Oat jar

5:3 Community Connection: Building a Supportive Vegan Network

In the heart of every movement lies the power of community. For those who walk the path of veganism, the journey is enriched by the connections made with like-minded individuals. A supportive vegan network can provide a sense of belonging, a space for sharing knowledge, and a wellspring of inspiration. This chapter delves into the essence of building a vegan community, offering insights and strategies to foster connections that support and sustain the vegan lifestyle.

The Foundation of a Vegan Community

The foundation of a vegan community is built on shared values and goals. It's a collective that thrives on empathy, compassion, and a commitment to a lifestyle that respects all forms of life. The Vegan Vanguard understands that to create lasting change, they must connect with others who share their vision for a kinder, more sustainable world.

Creating Spaces for Connection

Creating spaces where vegans can connect is vital for community building. These can be physical spaces like vegan cafes, farmers' markets, and community gardens, or virtual spaces such as online forums, social media groups, and webinars. These platforms allow individuals to exchange ideas, offer support, and celebrate the vegan lifestyle together.

Organizing Community Events

Events are the heartbeat of a community, bringing people together to learn, share, and grow. Organizing potlucks, cooking classes, film screenings, and speaker events are effective ways to engage the community. These gatherings can serve as a platform for education, activism, and the forging of new friendships.

Mentorship and Support Systems

For those new to veganism, the transition can be challenging. Establishing mentorship programs and support systems within the community can ease this process. Experienced vegans can offer guidance, answer questions, and provide resources to help newcomers navigate their journey with confidence.

Collaboration and Partnerships

Collaboration is the lifeblood of a thriving community. Forming partnerships with local businesses, non-profits, and educational institutions can amplify the community's reach and impact. These collaborations can lead to joint events, campaigns, and initiatives that further the cause of veganism.

Inclusivity and Diversity

A strong community is an inclusive one. Embracing diversity in all its forms—cultural, racial, economic—enriches the community and strengthens its foundation. It's about creating a welcoming environment where everyone's voice is heard and valued.

Advocacy and Outreach

A vegan community is not just inward-looking; it also reaches out to the wider public. Advocacy efforts such as leafleting, participating in fairs, and engaging in community service projects can raise awareness about veganism and its benefits for health, animals, and the environment.

Sustainability Initiatives

Sustainability initiatives are a natural extension of the vegan community's values. Projects like community composting, zero-waste workshops, and urban farming not only promote environmental stewardship but also bring people together for a common cause.

Celebrating Successes

Celebrating the successes and milestones of the community is crucial for maintaining momentum and morale. Whether it's the opening of a new vegan business, the adoption of plant-based options at local schools, or the passing of animal welfare legislation, every victory is a cause for celebration.

The Role of Storytelling

Storytelling is a powerful tool for community building. Sharing personal stories of transformation, the joys and challenges of vegan living, and the impact of collective action can inspire and motivate others. It's a way to

connect on a deeper level and to see the larger
narrative of the vegan movement unfold.

The Vegan Vanguard's Vision
The Vegan Vanguard envisions a world where
vegan communities are vibrant, active, and
influential. They see these communities as
catalysts for change, driving the shift towards a
more compassionate and sustainable future.
By building a supportive network, the Vegan
Vanguard is laying the groundwork for this
vision to become a reality.

Building a supportive vegan network is about
more than just sharing meals or attending
events; it's about creating a movement that is
rooted in compassion, driven by purpose, and
sustained by the bonds of community. It's a
testament to the power of collective action and
the belief that together, we can create a better
world.

Let this chapter serve as a guide for those
seeking to build or strengthen their vegan
community. Let it be a reminder that each
connection made, each event organized, and
each story shared is a step towards a more
compassionate, just, and sustainable world.

With passion, purpose, and the spirit of the Vegan Vanguard, we can build networks that not only support our lifestyle but also transform the world around us.

5:4 Legacy Recipes: Sharing Family Favorites and Creating New Traditions

In every culture, recipes are more than just instructions for preparing food; they are stories, memories, and traditions passed down through generations. They are the flavors of our childhoods, the aromas that wafted through our family kitchens, and the tastes that bring us back to moments long past. As members of the Vegan Vanguard, we honor these legacies while also forging new traditions that align with our compassionate lifestyle.

Honoring the Past

Legacy recipes are treasures, heirlooms that carry the essence of our heritage. They connect us to our roots, to the people who came before us, and to the experiences that shaped our families. Preserving these recipes is a way of honoring our ancestors, of keeping their memories alive, and of sharing their stories with new generations.

Adapting with Care

As we embrace a vegan lifestyle, we are often faced with the challenge of adapting these cherished recipes to fit our ethical choices. This adaptation is done with care and respect, seeking plant-based alternatives that maintain the integrity of the original dish. It's a creative process that involves trial and error, but the result is a new legacy that can be shared and celebrated.

Creating New Traditions

While we cherish the past, we also have the opportunity to create new traditions. These are recipes that will become the legacy we leave for future generations, dishes that reflect our values and the world we hope to build. They are a blend of the old and the new, combining time-honored techniques with innovative ingredients.

Recipes for Remembrance and Renewal

Here are some recipes that embody the spirit of legacy and tradition, each one a bridge between the past and the future.

Heirloom Lentil Stew
A hearty stew that pays homage to the
comforting dishes of our grandparents,
updated with plant-based ingredients.

Ingredients:
2 cups brown lentils, rinsed

1 large onion, diced

2 carrots, diced

2 celery stalks, diced

3 garlic cloves, minced

1 can diced tomatoes

6 cups vegetable broth

2 teaspoons thyme

2 bay leaves

Salt and pepper to taste

Fresh parsley for garnish

Instructions:
1. In a large pot, sauté onion, carrots, celery, and garlic until softened.
2. Add lentils, tomatoes, vegetable broth, thyme, and bay leaves.
3. Bring to a boil, then reduce heat and simmer until lentils are tender, about 30 minutes.
4. Season with salt and pepper. Garnish with fresh parsley before serving.

Modern Ratatouille

A vibrant dish that captures the essence of summer, this ratatouille is a celebration of vegetables and a nod to traditional French cooking.

Ingredients:
1 eggplant, sliced into rounds

2 zucchinis, sliced into rounds

2 yellow squashes, sliced into rounds

1 bell pepper, sliced

1 onion, sliced

3 tomatoes, sliced

3 tablespoons olive oil

2 garlic cloves, minced

1 teaspoon rosemary

Salt and pepper to taste

Instructions:
1. Preheat the oven to 375°F (190°C).
2. In a baking dish, arrange slices of eggplant, zucchini, squash, bell pepper, onion, and tomatoes in a spiral pattern.
3. Drizzle with olive oil and sprinkle with minced garlic, rosemary, salt, and pepper.
4. Cover with foil and bake for 40 minutes. Remove foil and bake for an additional 20 minutes until vegetables are tender.

Tips for Legacy Cooking

Document the Journey: Keep a journal or blog of your recipe adaptations and creations, documenting the process and the stories behind each dish.
Involve Family and Friends: Cooking is a communal activity. Involve loved ones in the

process of adapting and creating recipes, making it a shared experience.

Eat to Celebrate: Mark special occasions with your legacy recipes, making them a central part of your celebrations and gatherings.

The Vegan Vanguard's Commitment

The Vegan Vanguard's commitment to legacy recipes is a reflection of their dedication to a life of compassion and sustainability. It's about celebrating where we come from while being mindful of where we are going. It's about sharing meals that tell the stories of our past and our hopes for the future.

Legacy recipes are a vital part of our cultural fabric, connecting us to our history and to each other. As we adapt and create new traditions, we weave a richer tapestry that includes the best of what we've inherited and the best of what we aspire to be. Let these recipes be a source of comfort, joy, and inspiration, as we continue to cook with passion, purpose, and the spirit of the Vegan Vanguard.

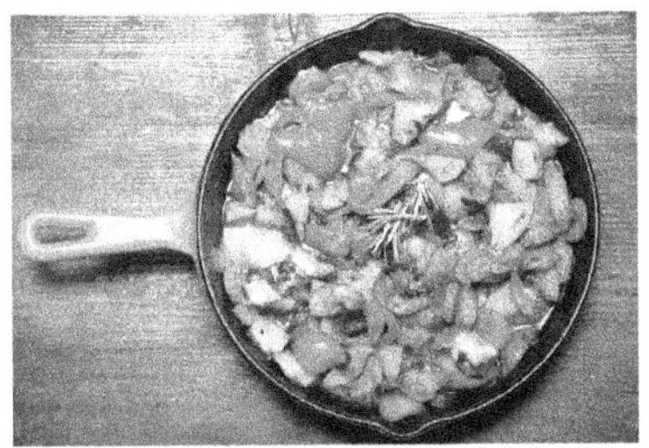

Ratatouille

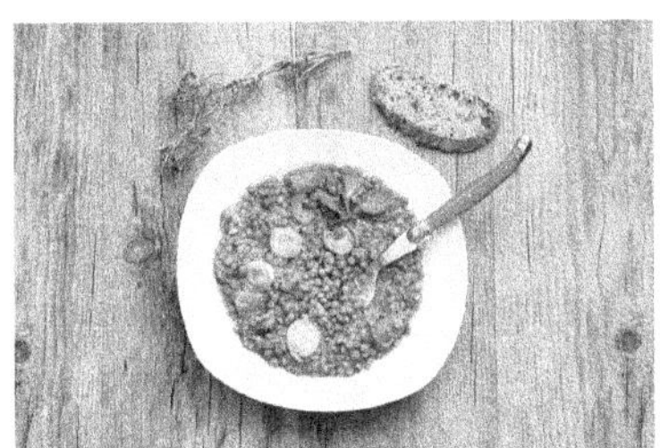

Lentil stew

CONCLUSION

As we turn the final page of **"The Vegan Vanguard**," we reflect on a journey that has been both enlightening and transformative. The concepts of compassion, sustainability, and innovation are interwoven throughout this book, which is more than just a compilation of chapters. It has been a guide, a companion, and a source of inspiration for those who seek to live with intention and purpose.

At the heart of the **Vegan Vanguard** beats a rhythm of change—a desire to create a world that is kinder, more just, and sustainable. Through the pages of this book, we have explored the many facets of veganism, from the food we eat to the choices we make every day. We have learned that being part of the Vanguard is not about perfection; it's about striving to make better choices, one step at a time.

Each chapter has added color and texture to our understanding of what it means to be vegan. We've delved into the richness of plant-based cuisine, the joy of sharing meals, and the importance of preserving the culinary legacies that connect us to our past. We've embraced the challenge of adapting traditional recipes and the creativity of inventing new ones, all while holding true to our ethical compass.

We've seen the strength that comes from community—the support, the shared experiences, and the collective wisdom that make our individual journeys richer and more meaningful. **The Vegan Vanguard** is not a solitary path but a shared voyage, where each of us contributes to the greater good.

Throughout this book, we've been reminded that living as a vegan is about more than diet—it's a holistic approach to life. It's about making conscious decisions that reflect our values, whether it's in the way we eat, the products we buy, or the causes we support. It's about living with purpose, passion, and an unwavering commitment to our principles.

As we close this chapter, let us view it not as an ending but as a beginning. Let this book be a call to action, a spark that ignites a flame of passion and purpose within each of us. Let us carry forward the spirit of the **Vegan Vanguard,** spreading its message through our actions and our words.

The legacy of the **Vegan Vanguard** is one that we write with every choice we make. It's a legacy of hope, of resilience, and of a belief that a better world is possible. It's a legacy that we will pass on to future generations, a testament to the power of living with compassion and conviction.

The Vegan Vanguard is more than just a book; it's a movement, a philosophy, and a way of life. It's a reminder that each of us has the power to make a difference, to be a force for good in the world. As we move forward, let us do so with the knowledge that we are part of something greater than ourselves—a vanguard for a brighter, more compassionate future.

Let us go forth with the passion of our convictions, the purpose of our actions, and the spirit of the Vegan Vanguard guiding us every step of the way. For in the end, we are not just vegans, we are vanguards, pioneers of a new dawn, and architects of a world where all beings can live in harmony.